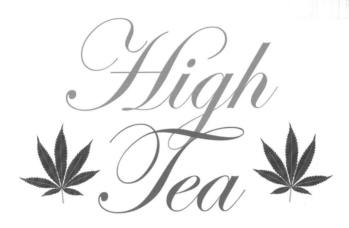

High Tea

All-Natural Cannabis Recipes for Relaxation and Wellness

SANDRA HINCHLIFFE
Author of *The Cannabis Spa at Home*

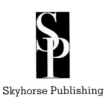

Skyhorse Publishing

Also by Sandra Hinchliffe

The Cannabis Spa at Home
CBD Every Day

Skyhorse Publishing books may be purchased in bulk at special discounts for sales promotion, corporate gifts, fund-raising, or educational purposes. Special editions can also be created to specifications. For details, contact the Special Sales Department, Skyhorse Publishing, 307 West 36th Street, 11th Floor, New York, NY 10018 or info@skyhorsepublishing.com.

Skyhorse® and Skyhorse Publishing® are registered trademarks of Skyhorse Publishing, Inc.®, a Delaware corporation.

Visit our website at www.skyhorsepublishing.com.

10 9 8 7 6 5 4 3 2 1

Library of Congress Cataloging-in-Publication Data is available on file.

Cover design by Laura Klynstra
Cover photo credit Sandra Hinchliffe

Paperback ISBN: 978-1-5107-5144-6
Ebook ISBN: 978-1-5107-1759-6

Printed in China

DEDICATION

To Chef Roxanna

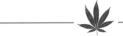

ACKNOWLEDGMENTS

Special thanks to my dear and bestest foraging pal, Janet; my husband, Greg; my agent, Rita Rosenkranz; and my editor at Skyhorse Publishing, Nicole Frail.

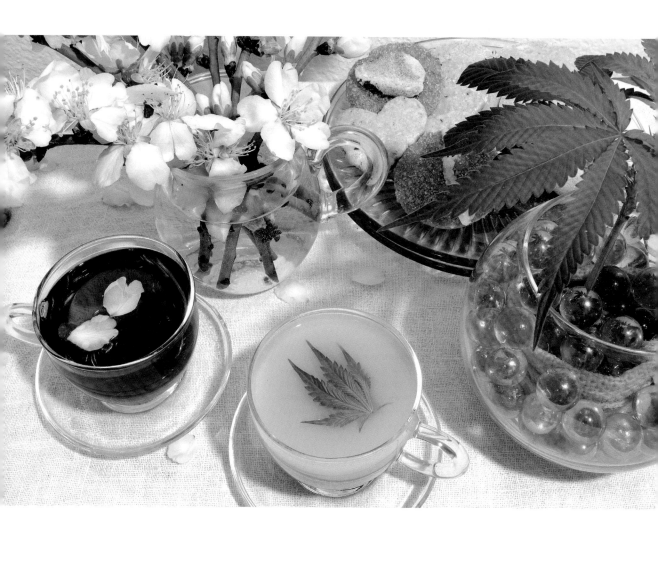

PREFACE

This book is intended for readers twenty-one and older.

The legality of the cannabis plant, as well as the other plants, possession, preparation, and consumption techniques of cannabis and other herbs varies by location—please consult your attorney for advice regarding the legal use of any plant. This book does not advocate unlawful behavior.

In addition, this book is not a replacement for the advice and diagnosis of a medical doctor—and nothing in this book should be considered medical advice. Please consult with your doctor regarding cannabis, other herbs, and your health. The recipes and suggestions in this book are not intended for pregnant or nursing mothers.

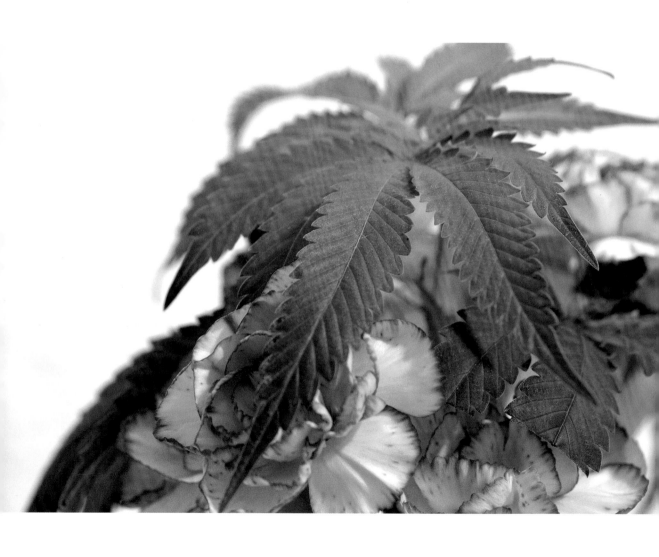

TABLE OF CONTENTS

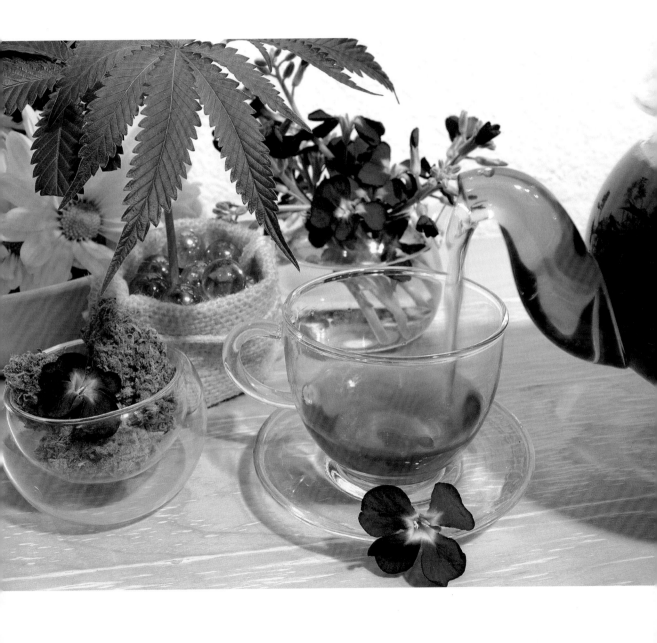

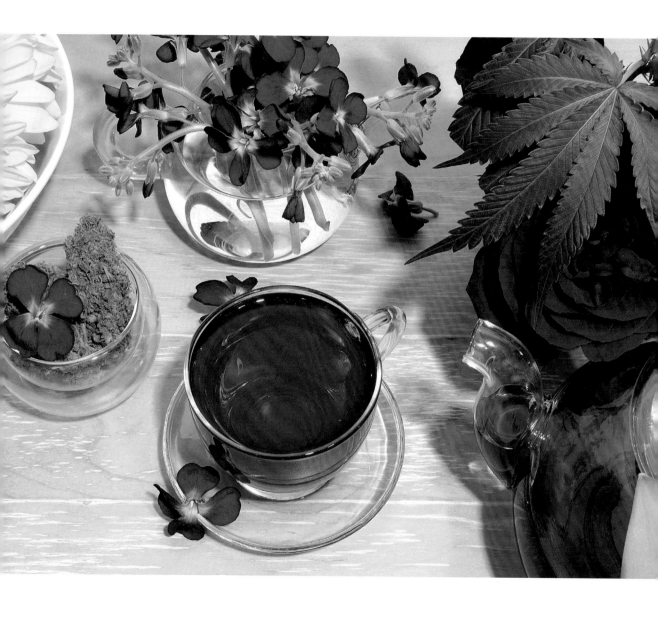

AN INTRODUCTION TO CANNABIS TEA-TIME AND THE ART OF CANNABIS TEA

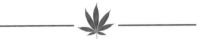

Why tea?

Teas, tisanes, broths, and bhangs are simple joys that can be prepared quickly and create flavor experiences, moods, and settings perfect for all the good vibrations the cannabis plant has to offer!

A Satisfying Experience: Cannabis Tea and Beverage

I believe that the best culinary cannabinoid experience is found in the form of teas, tisanes, and broths served with an herbal entourage, as well as creamy bhangs and beverages highly spiced or infused with bright, expansive flavors. These have a distinct advantage over cannabis cuisine; they generally have a faster onset, which is easier to titrate much like vaping cannabis, resulting in a positive and uplifting experience that will harness the power of CBD and THC along with other entourage chemistry, such as additional cannabinoids, monounsaturated fats, and the terpene chemistry of select herbs, fruits, and flowers.

Teas, tisanes, broths, and bhangs also do not lend themselves to overconsumption the way a snack food or entrée might. However, the cannabis beverages in this book can be paired with unmedicated small bites, pastries, or sweets that are complementary to the cannabis experience—and I recommend these types of pairings for the most satisfying experiences.

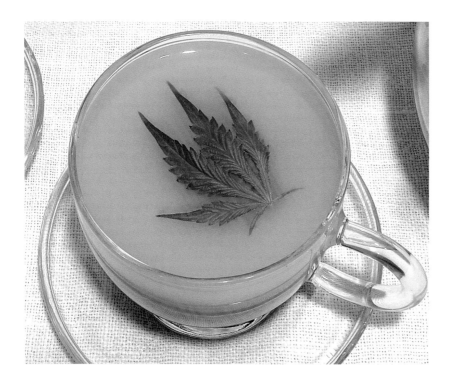

It's not surprising that bhang has been the preferred form of cannabis cuisine for thousands of years in India, where some traditions are deeply rooted in cannabis beverage consumption. The milky, lukewarm bhang made with whole cannabis and spices is a favorite and appropriate beverage for the Holi celebration and is openly sold by shops and vendors who cater to this cultural and spiritual tradition.

Infusing Cannabinoids into Beverages and Broths

Many know that the best cannabis infusions distribute the oily cannabinoids throughout liquids. This kind of robust infusion, known as

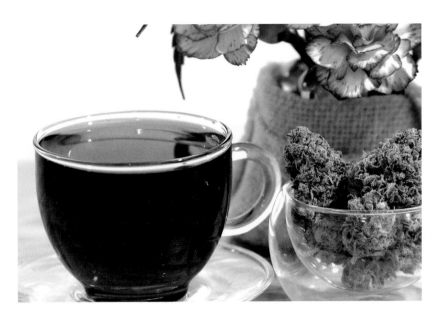

emulsification, is typical for cannabis beverages like bhang due to their heavy milk or nut-based preparation. In other types of beverages or broths, more often than not, the infusion of cannabinoids results in a floating layer of oil or resin on top of the beverage and a flavor that overpowers everything else.

Cannabinoids can only be extracted into fats or fat solvents that can then be infused into other things like beverages. You can't actually make a cannabinoid beverage or tea out of just water and cannabis flowers or concentrates and expect much more than floating resin that sticks to the pot or cup—unless you are juicing fresh cannabis, which is a completely different type of beverage. This is also why I think that alcohol-based cannabis tinctures are not ideal for beverages due to the cannabis oils sticking to the serviceware or cup.

Furthermore, cannabinoids need to be treated with heat to decarboxylate, or decarb, and become the active cannabinoids like CBD and the

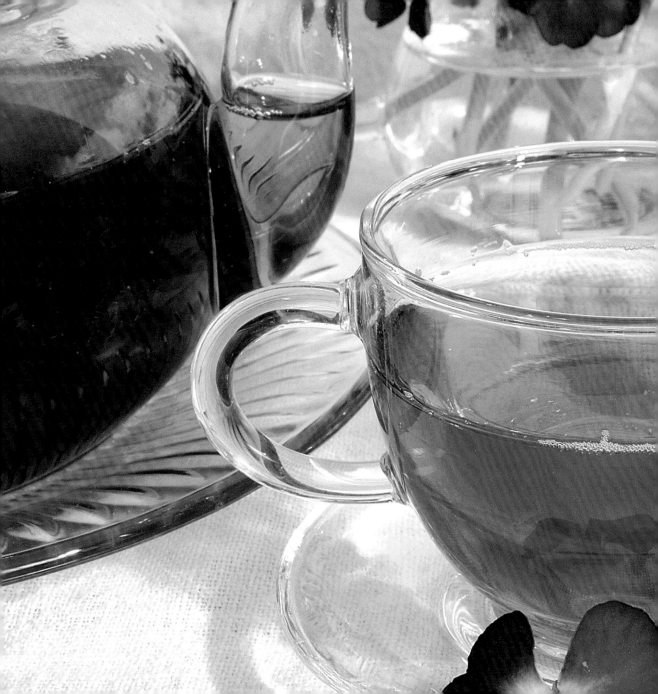

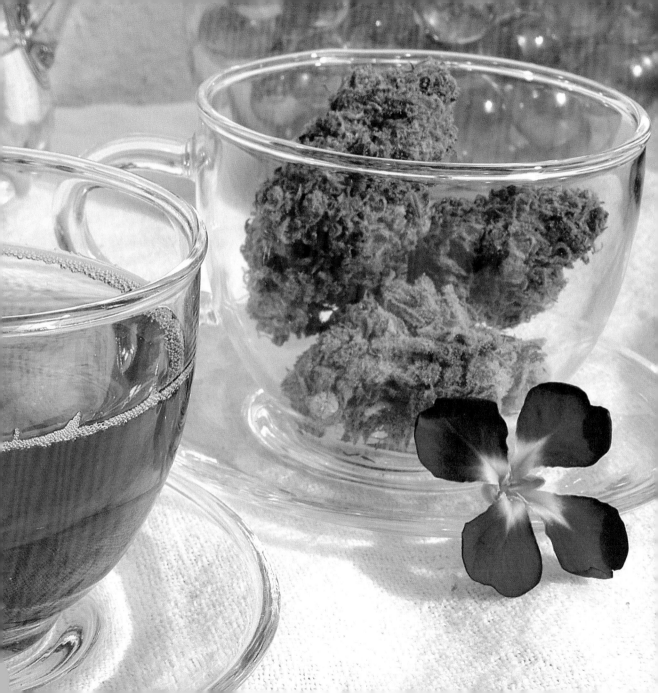

psychoactive cannabinoid THC if you desire the psychoactive effects. You may fully decarb, or even partially decarb—your preference. Cannabis may be consumed with very little to no decarboxylation for other health benefits, as well. For the purposes of our recipes, the extraction methods in this book are decarboxylated.

I offer to you three methods of cannabis infusion that have given the guests I have had the pleasure of serving the most flavorful and enjoyable experience in tea, tisane, broth, and bhang: The Cannabis Infusion Oil (page 11), the Tabletop Cannabis Infusion (page 33), and the Cannabis Milk Infusion for Bhang and Dessert Beverages (page 108) in chapter 4. These infusion recipes are explored in a variety of ways in the recipes that follow.

Dosing

Cannabis cuisine can be a wily, Wild West kind of experience for many people, both connoisseurs and new initiates, due to the powerful chemistry of THC as it passes through the liver and changes from delta-9 THC into 11-hydroxy-THC—the latter being more psychedelic than the former for many. I don't think I know a single cannabis consumer who hasn't had at least one negative experience with cannabis cuisine due to its unpredictability in many instances. And while CBD is a more gentle way to experience cannabis, especially for first-time consumers, in both instances with CBD or THC, many people have a better experience if this is absorbed mostly sublingually. Beverage is an excellent way to enjoy cannabinoids in this manner.

I'm often asked about accurate and effective dosing of cannabinoids. I know that without lab testing, there is no such thing as a completely accurate dosage. You can find calculators online and recommendations by top chefs may be quite helpful, but only lab testing is precise.

The best method for precise milligram counts is to purchase a cannabis product from a legal dispensary that has been tested by a lab and contains the milligram content on the packaging or a percentage of cannabinoids by weight so that you can calculate the milligrams as accurately as possible. Simple enough—you put the whole thing into the Cannabis Infusion Oil recipe in this chapter and then divide it into servings of *x* (your desired amount) milligrams of cannabinoids. This is the most accurate way of confirming the exact amount of cannabinoids you are consuming or serving to other people, apart from taking your final infusion oil to have it tested by a cannabis lab.

You can also follow this formula in a similar way using the Tabletop Cannabis Infusion (page 33) or the Cannabis Milk Infusion for Bhang and Dessert Tea (page 108).

My formulas for calculating cannabinoid milligrams in the recipes that I make use lab-tested cannabis products with the measurement in percentages of cannabinoids per weight, and looks like this:

X% × decimal gram weight = X decimal gram weight

To calculate Y milligrams, multiply the X decimal gram weight by 1000.
X decimal gram weight × 1000 = Y milligrams

Example: 1 gram of cold water hashish tests at 56% THC and 3% CBD.
56% × 1 = 0.56 and 3% × 1 = 0.03
0.56 × 1000 = 560 milligrams of THC per 1 gram weight
0.03 × 1000 = 30 milligrams of CBD per 1 gram weight

Example: Calculate the milligrams of cannabinoids in half a gram of oil or resin with 83% CBD and 0.30% THC
83% × 0.50 = 0.415
0.30 × 0.50 = 0.0015
0.415 × 1000 = 415 milligrams of CBD per 0.50 gram weight
0.0015 × 1000 = 1.5 milligrams of THC per 0.50 gram weight

Example: Calculate the milligrams of three different lab-tested hash concentrates and oils to combine into one recipe, such as the Cannabis Infusion Oil recipe (page 11):

    1 gram of hash oil extract is 55% THC or CBD
    + 1 gram of sifted hash 47% THC or CBD
    + 1 gram of kief 38% THC or CBD
    55 + 47 + 38 = 140

Divide by the number of grams (3, in this case) to calculate the average percentage of THC in all 3 grams combined.

    140 ÷ 3 = 46.67, or 46.67% of the weight of these three grams of cannabis concentrate is THC or CBD.

To calculate the milligrams, which will be contained in the final recipe:

    46.63 7% × 3 = 1.4001
    1.4001 × 1000 = 1400.1 total milligrams of THC or CBD when these 3 grams are combined into one recipe.

That said, many people reading this book are going to work with raw, cured cannabis flowers or even trim they have grown at home. I've always been an eyeball chef when it comes to homegrown. I know that when I've got a gram of top-shelf cannabis flower (with an estimated 18% or more THC, CBD, or a combination of both, based on my vaping experience with the flowers), I'm going to have about ten to fifteen servings of cannabinoids if I am serving tea to cannabis newbies and at least four or more servings for more experienced cannabis connoisseurs. My rule of thumb for serving myself or others has always been: whatever amount it takes in the vape for one session is the amount I'll put in a cup of tea or broth for myself or those I am serving. It's been a standard for me that has, so far, averted cannabis culinary disaster when it is impossible to make calculations based on known percentages of cannabinoids.

However, I do prefer exact measure whenever possible; and I recommend the lab-tested concentrated cannabis products because they create superior infusions that work beautifully with the tea, tisane, bhang, and broth recipes that follow. The less fragrant and more clean the oil extraction is, the better it will perform in a wide variety of recipes. Many of the tea, tisane, and broth formulations in this book have delicate flavors and terpene infusions designed to work best with clean cannabis oil concentrates used in the cannabis infusion recipes here.

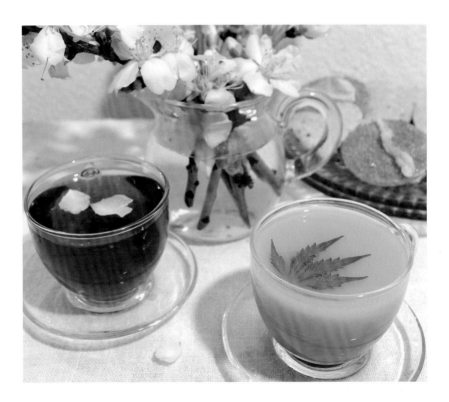

How much "high" to serve?

In my experience, and that of the guests whom I have had the pleasure of serving cannabis-infused tea, the typical onset of euphoria and medicinal effects, using my cannabis infusion formulations, is about fifteen to thirty minutes on an empty stomach, and no more than forty-five on a full stomach. As with anything, your mileage may vary, and you should always wait at least two hours after consuming cannabis to determine your sobriety before consuming more. That sounds like a long time, but patience is always going to be the better bargain, especially for cannabis beginners. I'm fairly certain, though, that you are going to be pleased with how fast-acting these beverage recipes are for most people.

The THC and CBD dosing I follow when serving others looks something like this:

- Microdosing: 2 milligrams or fewer
- Beginners: 2–5 milligrams
- Occasional Consumers: 5–10 milligrams
- Experienced Consumers: 10–20 milligrams
- Frequent Consumers: 15–50 milligrams
- Gurus: 50 milligrams or more

This is **per serving**. Servings should be spaced one to three hours before consuming more if you're starting with the maximum dose recommended. Other cannabinoids can be dosed in a similar manner. For example, CBD doesn't have much, if any, psychoactive effects like THC, but it may induce more drowsiness at higher doses.

One of my favorite ways to enjoy cannabis-infused tea is two or three cups at 5 milligrams of THC or CBD each. I find this to be very sensible in social gatherings. However, I have had as much as 90 milligrams of THC in one very powerful bhang! I don't suggest this unless you are

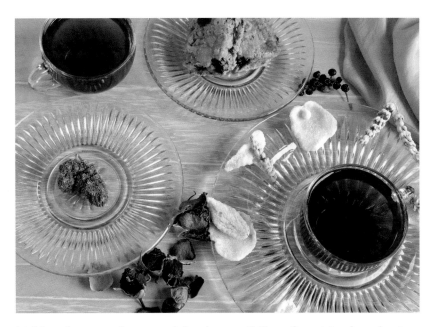

highly tolerant and prepared for the possibility of a spiritual awakening. I consume cannabis almost daily for the chronic pain that accompanies autoimmune disease and remain very sensitive to the effects even after all this time. Remember that we are all different and experience this herb in ways unique to us. Part of the discovery process that unfolds as we partake in the blessings of this herb is finding the cozy spot—the perfect entourage of cannabis constituents in a dosage amount that feels good! I hope you are ready to feel good, too!

The Cannabis Infusion Oil

My Cannabis Infusion Oil recipe creates a very concentrated cannabis oil that is emulsifiable in a hot liquid. It's also high in monounsaturated oleic acids, which have been shown to have positive benefits for mood

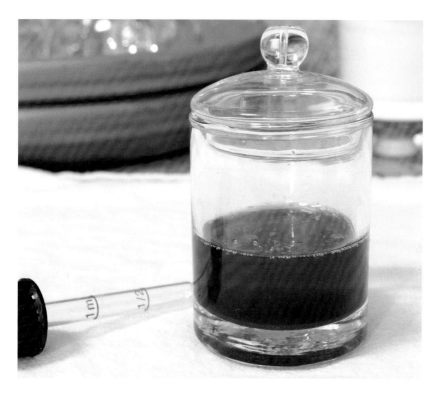

management in some clinical studies.[1] And that's just the kind of fat chemistry we need to create a satisfying experience with cannabis.

For most teas, tisanes, and broths, we will want to create an emulsification of these fats and cannabinoids that does not overwhelm a clear liquid

1   C Lawrence Kien; Janice Y Bunn; Connie L Tompkins; Julie A Dumas; Karen I Crain; David B Ebenstein; Timothy R Koves; Deborah M Muoio (2013) "Substituting dietary monounsaturated fat for saturated fat is associated with increased daily physical activity and resting energy expenditure and with changes in mood" *The American Journal of Clinical Nutrition* 97 (4): 689–697. https://www.ncbi.nlm.nih.gov/pubmed/23446891

and make it oily or heavy. This same Cannabis Infusion Oil recipe can be used in any beverage you would like to infuse with cannabis. This infusion oil can be gently swirled in the cup or bowl or emulsified with a whisk. It's also a shelf-stable and convenient way to prepare any cannabis beverage or broth quickly.

Cannabinoids concentrated in monounsaturated fats and phosphatidylcholines from sunflower lecithin are the foundation of our cannabis infusion symphony. To this end, the best Cannabis Infusion Oil is made from concentrated cannabinoids using hash oils, rosins, or CO_2 extractions and very little base oil so that the final amount of the oil used in each serving is very small—0.50 milliliters or even fewer.

The Cannabis Infusion Oil Ingredients

The basic infusion oil that will work in almost all the recipes in this book is shelf-stable and contains two ingredients to infuse the cannabinoids into beverages: rice bran oil (or coconut oil, or *Camellia oleifera* seed oil) and liquid sunflower lecithin. The final infusion oil that you create will be highly concentrated with cannabinoids, and you will need very small amounts for each of the recipes. Your clear beverages will remain clear, not oily or heavy. The taste will be quite mild if you are using very clean, concentrated cannabis oils to create the infusion oil, as well. Doses can then be measured in small amounts that emulsify into warm and hot liquids using a tea whisk or other small beverage whisk.

Rice Bran Oil and Coconut Oil

Rice bran oil is neutral in flavor and available in most Asian and natural foods markets. It's a lovely oil to use for infusing beverages with cannabinoids that will give excellent results—it's high in oleic acids, shelf-stable and temperature-stable, and free of all major allergens when produced in a dedicated factory. It has the advantage of being high in γ-oryzanol, which

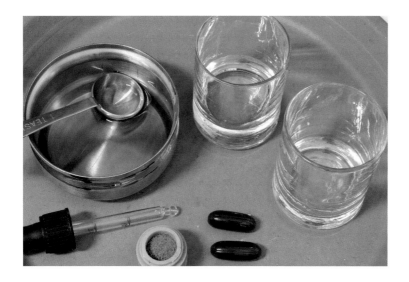

has some purported benefits for menopause and cholesterol issues.[2] It is the oil of choice to have on hand if you will be serving a variety of people or if you have allergies or sensitivities to nut-based oils.

If you'd like to use coconut oil as your base oil, this is also a shelf-stable oil with many great nutritional properties that may impart a mild or slight coconut flavor in beverages you include it in. I would recommend coconut oil for use with the milky cannabis teas and bhang recipes for the best flavor and texture. Coconut oil is also free of major allergens when it is produced in a dedicated factory that does not also process nuts.

Camellia oleifera seed oil

If the name Camellia looks familiar to you, that's because *Camellia oleifera* is related to the *Camellia sinensis*, otherwise known as the tea plant that

---

2   Patel, M and S N Naik. "Gamma-oryzanol from rice bran oil—A review." *Journal of Scientific and Industrial Research* Vol. 63 July 2004 pp 569–578. http://nopr. niscair.res.in/bitstream/123456789/5457/1/JSIR%2063(7)%20569–578.pdf

gives us the wide variety of black, green, and white teas we're familiar with. Your cup of tea, no matter what kind, always comes from the leaves and buds of the *Camellia sinensis var sinensis* or *var assamica* plant.

Camellia oleifera is a sister plant that produces a seed that is cold-pressed for its thin oil high in monounsaturated fats and oleic acid. *Camellia oleifera* tea seed oil is one of the lightest and least "oily" of all oils. Cannabis Infusion Oil made with this oil is my personal favorite for serving at my tea table due to its very subtle floral and fruity fragrance, which creates a pleasant-tasting cannabis oil extraction.

Although I have found that *Camellia oleifera* tea seed oil really shines as an oil base for the cannabinoids in these recipes, those with tree nut allergies may want to consult their physician before experimenting with this oil. *Camellia oleifera* does produce a fruit that opens up to release seeds that are not generally classified as nuts—but it is still worth checking with your doctor on this one if you have nut allergies.

Don't confuse *Camellia oleifera* tea seed oil with camelina seed oil or tea tree oil—these are both very different oils. Make sure that the oil you purchase is 100 percent culinary-grade *Camellia oleifera* tea seed oil. Many Asian markets carry this as a specialty oil or you can order it online.

Sunflower Seed Lecithin

Liquid sunflower seed lecithin is an allergy-friendly form of lecithin free of eggs and soy. It makes a pretty good emulsifier for cannabis-infused tea without affecting the flavor or body of the beverage. It's also chockfull of phosphatidylcholines, which have numerous nutritional benefits for the brain and nervous system.[3] It's a fabulous complement to the chemistry of cannabinoids.

---

3   Fernstrom, John D. "Can nutrient supplements modify brain function?" *The American Journal of Clinical Nutrition* June 2000 vol. 71 no. 6 1669s-1673s 1–3 http://ajcn.nutrition.org/content/71/6/1669s.full.pdf+html

The Cannabis Infusion Oil Recipes

Cannabis Infusion Oil with Concentrated Cannabinoids (Hash Oil, Rosin, Hashish)

Using this recipe, you will create an emulsifiable infusion oil using lab-tested, pure cannabis concentrates with very little fragrance. This shelf-stable recipe will keep for months in your cabinet but is best used within three to four months. For the best flavor in tea, tisane, broth, or any beverage, concentrate the cannabinoids in the final infusion oil so that the final serving size is 0.50 milliliters or even fewer, which is ideal. This recipe can be doubled, tripled, or more using this basic small-batch formula.

Preparation:

1. Sterilize the glass jar or bottle that you will be using to store your final Cannabis Infusion Oil in boiling water, dry, and set aside.
2. The best way to produce this oil is with two very small stainless steel dishes or pans set up together as a double-boiler. The dish or pan below

30 milliliters (2 tablespoons) base oil (rice bran oil, coconut oil, camellia seed oil)

3 grams (3 milliliters) waxy/liquid sunflower lecithin (Consistency depends on brand.)

1–2 grams or more of any THC or CBD cannabis concentrate (Low fragrance, clean varieties work best.)

Glass storage container

Eyedropper or syringe with milliliters marked on the glass for measuring serving sizes with ease

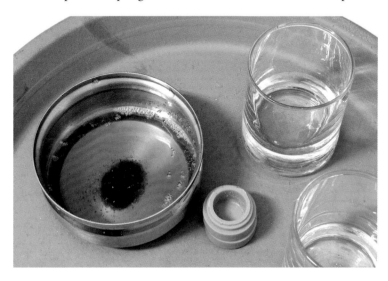

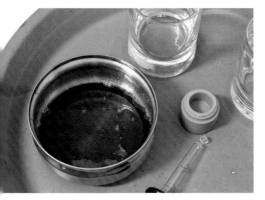

contains water and the dish or pan on top contains the base oil and hashish. Heat on medium to low for 1 hour, making sure the water does not boil off completely. Add more water, if necessary. This will decarboxylate the cannabinoids in the cannabis concentrate—a necessary step to create a psychoactive oil. Alternatively, you could place the oil dish or pan in your oven at 350°F (177°C) for 1 hour to decarboxylate, if you prefer. The double-boiler method will have a cleaner flavor, so this is the one I recommend.

3. After you have completed the decarboxylation of the cannabinoids, add the sunflower lecithin while the oil is still hot and dissolve it thoroughly into the hot oil. Allow this to cool for 15 to 20 minutes and then transfer into the clean glass storage jar that you will be using. To thoroughly remove the oil from the dish or pan, use a small silicone spatula and scrape the insides.

4. Your oil is now ready for the calculator. You will now calculate your final cannabinoid milligram content and label your jar with this information. Calculate following the dosage calculation, which was explained in the dosing section of this chapter (see page 6).

Here is an example calculation for this recipe:
- Approximately 33 milliliters in the final oil =
  - 30 milliliters of base oil
  - 3 milliliters or 3 grams of sunflower lecithin
  - 1 gram of cannabis concentrate

In this example, the gram of cannabis concentrate added to the oil contained 780 milligrams of THC and 30 milligrams of CBD (your numbers will differ from this example).

This cannabis infusion oil example makes approximately 66 (0.50-milliliter) servings. Each serving size is 0.50 milliliter with approximately 12 milligrams of THC and 0.45 milligrams of CBD.

The Cannabis Flower Infusion Oil

This recipe is really for people who want to incorporate the whole natural cannabis flavor and fragrance into their final beverage or broth. Don't be afraid of the natural fragrance and flavor of cannabis; in some recipes, like a traditional bhang beverage, it can work quite well. If you'd like to try your hand at a flavorful cannabis-infused oil that uses cannabis flowers, this is the recipe I use when pairing with beverages where the fragrance and flavor of whole cannabis flowers is desired. I think it works nicely in some savory broths in chapter 3, as well.

This whole flower formulation will introduce more oil into the final beverage or broth than the highly concentrated Cannabis Infusion Oil recipe formulated with cannabis concentrates, so it is best reserved for beverage or broths where this is desirable. Makes 4 to 10 servings or more. This infusion oil recipe is shelf-stable at room temperature and can be doubled, tripled, or more using this basic small-batch formula.

15 milliliters (1 tablespoon) base oil (rice bran oil, coconut oil, camellia seed oil)

2 grams (2 milliliters) waxy/liquid sunflower lecithin

1 gram or as much as 2 grams of top-shelf cannabis flower (18% or more cannabinoids), finely ground

Small glass storage container, if needed

Eyedropper or syringe with milliliters marked on the glass for measuring serving sizes with ease

Preparation:

1. You'll probably be using this oil right away, but if that's not the case, proceed as you would in the first recipe for the concentrated oil and sterilize a glass container to store the final oil.

2. This oil has the best flavor when it is produced using a double-boiler method. Two small stainless steel dishes or pans can be set up in this manner to decarboxylate and extract the cannabinoids from the plant material. Fill the bottom pan with water, and place the pan containing the base oil and the ground cannabis flowers on top of this. Heat on low for 1 hour, making sure the water does

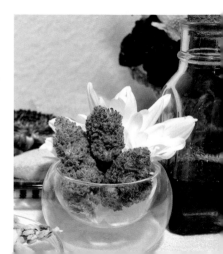

not boil off completely. Remove from the heat and allow this to cool before squeezing as much of the oil as possible from the ground cannabis material.

3. Warm the oil and dissolve the sunflower lecithin into it. Allow this to cool, and it is ready to use.
4. Your oil is now ready to portion into servings.

Let's take a look at an example recipe calculation using 1 gram of cannabis flowers with 18% THC:

- Approximately 16 milliliters of the final oil =
  - 15 milliliters of base oil
  - 2 grams or 2 milliliters of sunflower lecithin

(After the plant material has been strained out, measure the oil to ensure the exact milliliters—some of the oil will inevitably stick to the plant material even when it is strained well.)

So, 180 milligrams of THC in 16 milliliters of oil and sunflower lecithin = 16 (1-milliliter) servings of oil with approximately 11.25 milligrams of THC per serving. (Your final numbers will vary.)

Obtain the Best Results with Cannabis Infusion Oil

Whether you're making a hot or cold cannabis beverage or broth, the most effective ways to infuse and emulsify the Cannabis Infusion Oil recipe into any liquid are to:

- Always stir the oil well before taking it up into the measured eye dropper or syringe to portion into the recipes.
- Start the infusion in a hot liquid. The best result is obtained when the oil is first added to the serviceware like a teapot, pitcher, tureen, or mug, and the hot liquid is slowly poured into them while whisking the liquid into the oil vigorously. Then you can

serve. If the final beverage or broth is a cold liquid, start with a small amount of it heated until steaming in a pan on the stove, vigorously whisk the liquid into the serviceware that you have portioned the cannabis oil into, and then add to the cool or cold liquid while whisking again before serving cool or cold over ice.

- I like to use small whisks for cups and larger whisks for teapots or tureens. Bamboo tea whisks designed for matcha work nicely, as well, to emulsify and effectively infuse the oil into warm or hot liquids. But any kitchen whisk will do.

- While not always necessary for hot liquids, for the most effective emulsification without thickening or changing the flavor, you should whisk into the liquid a pinch per serving of very pure, food-grade Senegal acacia gum fiber before whisking the liquid into the oil. You should always do this if you're making cold beverages. I recommend Heather's Tummy Fiber as a reliable, organic, acacia gum brand that works well in every recipe in this book that calls for it, but any comparable source of Senegal acacia gum powder may be used.

Try a quick cuppa right now using the Cannabis Infusion Oil recipe!

You've selected and made your infusion oil, so now it's time to taste it. Let's start with something really simple: a cup and your favorite bagged tea. This recipe can serve one or more people.

Preparation:

1. Bring the water to a boil in your serviceware and portion the Cannabis Infusion Oil to your cups. Add the bags to the hot water and steep for 1 to 3 minutes. Remove the bags, and add a pinch of Senegal acacia gum

1 or more servings of Cannabis Infusion Oil
1 pot of boiling water, premeasured for your cup or mug
1 bag or more of your favorite tea
Pinch of Senegal acacia gum (optional)
Your favorite tea cups or mugs

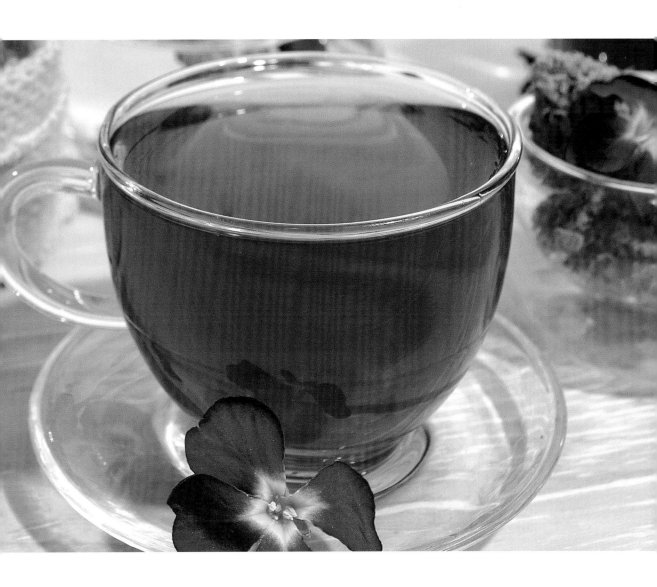

powder, if desired. Tea bags or loose tea should not come into contact with the oil because they will absorb it.

2. Slowly pour the tea into the cups and whisk the liquid into the oil vigorously with a whisk.

3. Serve plain or with sweeteners, milks, or lemon, and enjoy. Tea should be served immediately or whisked again if service is delayed.

4. If you'd like to serve several people from one teapot, you may add the number of Cannabis Infusion Oil servings directly to the teapot and then slowly pour the hot liquid in to the pot while whisking, and serve.

Gong Fu versus Western Brewing

So far, you have learned how to prepare Western-style tea infused with cannabis, such as your favorite bagged tea or a robustly steeped pot of tea, but by far, the Gong Fu method is my favorite way to prepare cannabis-infused tea. This method will produce a cup that is always true to the flavors and clarity of the tea.

Gong Fu, the method of tea preparation originating in China, is the superior way to prepare tea, and the difference is quite notable in the taste, body, and fragrance. Far from being too formal for everyday tea enjoyment like the traditional Western tea table, or low tea, with its immaculate tablewares, sparkle, and lace, Gong Fu is a very down-to-earth way of enjoying the best that tea has to offer and does not require a plethora of elaborate and expensive settings or teaware. Gong Fu is so simple and pure, it is quite possibly the most elegant way to prepare cannabis-infused tea to impress or enjoy everyday.

Gong Fu has a lot of surprising elements, such as its preparation on a wet table or tray to accommodate the rinsing of the teas, warming of the cups and teaware, and multiple infusions of generous portions of loose tea leaves. Gong Fu preparation exclusively uses loose leaf teas, and in a much greater quantity than Western-style brewing methods—approximately

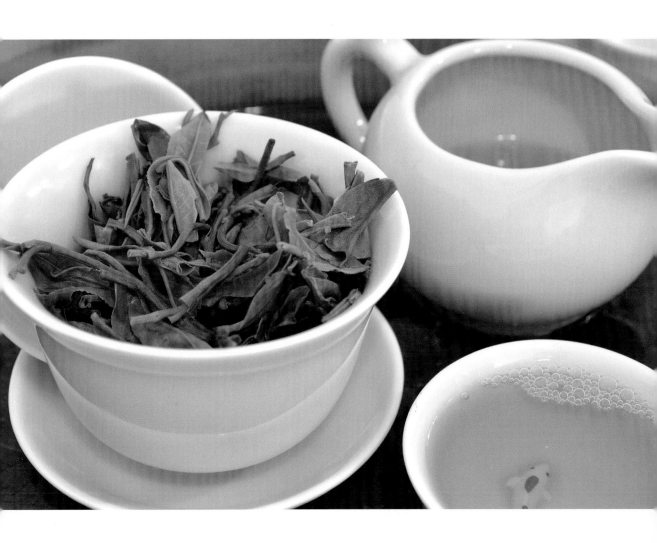

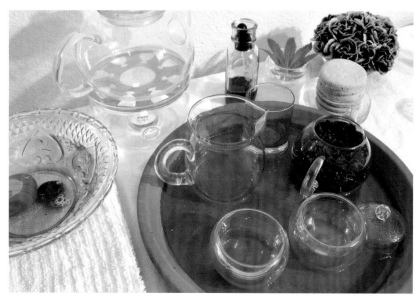

On the left, about 2 teaspoons (or 2–4 grams) of tea for a Western-style brew, and on the right, more than 5 teaspoons (or about 6–10 grams) of tea for Gong Fu preparation.

three to four times as much tea. And these are steeped with less water, multiple times, for 5 to 20 seconds depending on the tea.

Cannabis-Infused Tea Gong Fu Style

The most basic teaware for Gong Fu preparation consists of a *gaiwan* (a ceramic bowl with a lid) or a small pot; a *chahai*, *gong dao bei*, or serving pitcher; *pinming*, shallow *chawan*, or small tasting cups; along with a Gong Fu drainage tray or wet trays and a basin for waste water after warming the teaware and rinsing the tea. These teawares can be as humble or exotic as you desire, and you can find many beautiful Gong Fu tray and tea sets to purchase from tea shops and online. However, a simple, shallow clay dish and borosilicate glassware will produce the same immaculate flavors of an expensive Gong Fu set.

Flavor, body, and fragrance are sometimes limiting factors when infusing anything with cannabis—and that's what makes Gong Fu tea preparation a fantastic way to prepare cannabis-infused tea. You will brew multiple times, adding only 1 or 2 drops of the Cannabis Infusion Oil to the small cups used for Gong Fu tea service each time the tea is steeped and poured. The technique is simple: draw up the desired amount of oil into a measured eyedropper as shown here and add to your cup 1 or 2 drops per serving, finishing the dose through multiple steeps and servings. Gong Fu preparation and service requires no whisking like some other beverages due to the small drops of oil used in each cup. The drops may be swirled in the cup while drinking.

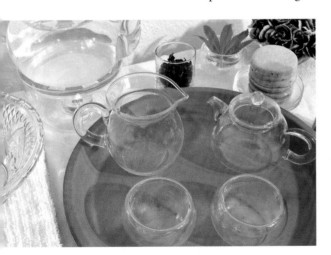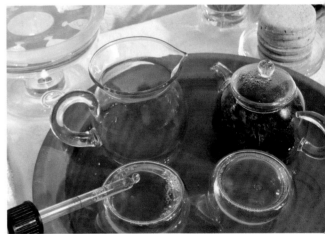

Step-By-Step Gong Fu Cannabis-Infused Tea

Depending on the Gong Fu tea service you have selected, such as a grated drainage table designed for Gong Fu service—or the most basic setup with a shallow clay dish, borosilicate teaware, and a glass basin with your favorite stones or ceramic tea pets—your steps in the preparation of this cannabis-infused tea may vary. The steps here are the essential steps for a Gong Fu experience.

1. Begin by heating a large pot of spring water or filtered tap water to the appropriate temperature recommended for the tea you will be using. Slightly mineralized water from a spring or filtered tap will give the best flavor, body, and fragrance. I would encourage you to experiment with water, as there are no hard rules on this! I've had a lovely Gong Fu session using very fresh rainwater, but your success with this will depend on the tea you select.

2. When the hot water is ready, pour some over and into the teaware to warm them. After a minute or so, dump the water from the teapot or gaiwan into the water refuse basin or tray with your stones or over your tea pet. Fill the teapot or gaiwan with the fresh tea leaves after you empty the hot water.

3. Empty all the hot water warming the teaware into the basin, and add fresh hot water to the tea leaves in the teapot or gaiwan, paying special attention to the ratio of water to tea. For example, 4–6 teaspoons (or about 5–7 grams) of tea leaves should be steeped in approximately 1 cup (or about 240 milliliters) of water each time the leaves are infused.

4. After 5 to 10 seconds of steeping, you will then pour this first infusion into the serving pitcher and cups to warm them again, and then dump this first infusion into the basin or your tea tray with grates and basin—do not drink it. The first steep of Gong Fu tea is not meant for drinking; the first steep warms your teaware, washes your leaves, and awakens them, but is never for drinking. Your stones or tea pet are given

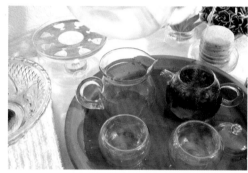

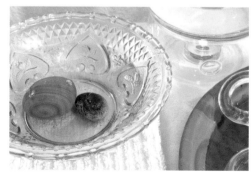

As you can see here, I have selected some pretty stones from the beach for my basin, but you can use any stones or even a ceramic tea pet sold for this purpose in most proper tea shops.

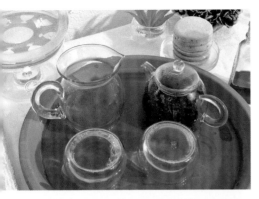

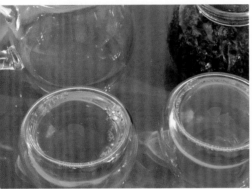

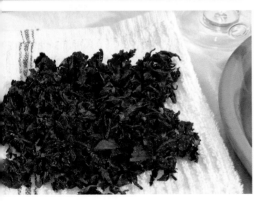

this steep, and later you can use the waste water for your cannabis garden!

5. Now you're ready to prepare the tea for drinking. Add the same amount of hot water you used to make the first infusion into your teapot or gaiwan, and let this steep 5 to 30 seconds, depending on what is recommended for the type of tea you're using. Feel free to experiment with different steeping times to experience the various flavor aspects of the tea that come out based on temperature and steep timings. However, the maximum for Gong Fu steeping is typically around 20 seconds, with most teas in about the 10 second range. After the tea has steeped, pour it into the serving pitcher and then use the pitcher to fill each cup.

6. After you have poured the tea into the individual cups, your premeasured dropper of Cannabis Infusion Oil should be filled with the desired dose for this tea session. Use the dropper to add only 1 or 2 drops to each cup, and then serve the tea.

7. The number of infusions you can get out of your tea leaves will depend on the type of tea you're using. Typically, you will get five or more infusions from the leaves, and some teas like oolong will steep up to twenty times! Although Gong Fu tea preparation uses much more tea than the typical Western-style brewing method, it is indeed economical due to the multiple times it can be steeped. You can repeat the infusion steps now, adding a drop of the Cannabis Infusion Oil to each cup before it is served. If the tea liquor goes cold in your serving pitcher before it can be added to the cups, give this to your tea stones or tea pet in the basin and prepare hot tea again. Remember

to increase the steeping time by a few seconds for each sequential steep for the best flavor.

8. If you aren't able to finish the leaves through the maximum number of infusions they can deliver, don't throw them away. Spread them out on a clean, porous clay dish or tea towel and allow them to air dry on your tea table until later or even the next day. When you're ready to work with them again, put them back in the pot and continue repeating the steeping process. There's no need to rinse or awaken these leaves again after you have done it in the first infusion.

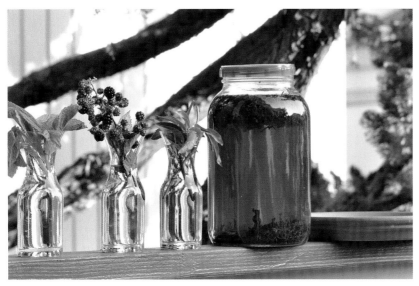

Here's a tip for working with the leftover tea leaves after your Gong Fu session: Spread the leaves on a clay or ceramic plate and fully dry them in the sun. Store them after drying and use generous amounts for infusing as sun tea. At this point, your high quality tea leaves will have delivered their maximum number of infusions and you can now send them to your compost pile.

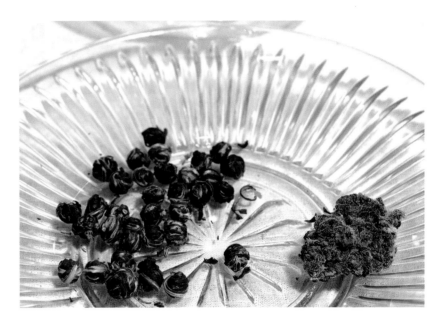

Artful Cannabis and Tea Pairings

The rule of thumb for serving the most desirable flavors and fragrances in cannabis-infused tea is the pairing of the natural tea flavors to the cannabis product you have on hand. The lighter the fragrance and flavor of the cannabis product, such as a clean extracted hash oil, the more subtle it is in very delicate teas. The richer in cannabis flavor and fragrance, like a whole cannabis flower infusion, the more delicious it is in rich, toasted, or smoky teas—like very toasty jasmine, smoked black teas, genmaicha, or twig teas. However, the flavor of cannabis does have a tendency to overpower the flavors of tea—you will never go wrong with a very clean cannabis extraction, and this is what I recommend for working with both tea and tisane.

Smoky Dragon Blossom Tea Tasting

This ethereal cannabis tea tasting uses a Fujian jasmine pearl tea that has been generously layered with jasmine flowers over the course of many days, rolled, and then roasted dry. There are different methods used to produce these pearl teas, and you'll want to select the one with a toasty flavor. This type of toasted jasmine pearl tea will be browner in color and golden in the cup. It's a high-quality tea that will typically steep two or more times with variations on the flavor each time. I prepare this tea using the Gong fu method for the best flavor. Makes many servings!

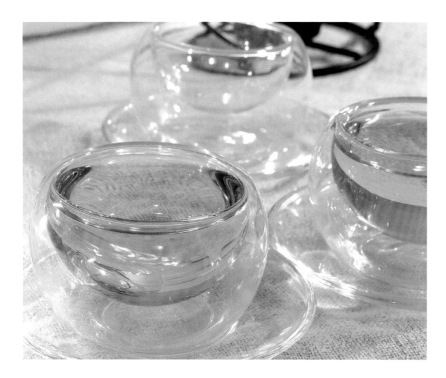

Preparation and Service:

1. Prepare the Cannabis Infusion Oil, and measure the desired dose for as many people as you are serving. Set this with the rest of your Gong fu table. Arrange flowers, your basin with stones or tea pet, cups, pots, trays, and other serviceware. This tea is also delicious when served with the Arrowroot Tea Biscuit from chapter 5 (page 138). Have those ready to serve with the tea before you begin, if desired.

2. The amount of tea you will be using will depend on how many people you will be serving. To serve two people, your tea-to-water ratio will look something like this: 6–8 teaspoons (or about 8 grams) of tea and 6–8 ounces (or 200–240 milliliters) of water, each steep heated to 190°F (or 87°C).

3. Prepare the first steep and hold in the pot or gaiwan for about 5 seconds. Then fill your cups and serving pitcher to warm them, and then dump into your basin with stones or over your tea pet on your Gong Fu tray.

4. Prepare the second steep for about 10 seconds, pour into your serving pitcher, and then into the cups. Add 1 or 2 drops of the Cannabis Infusion Oil into each cup and serve.

5. Repeat step four as many times as you would like—feel free to experiment with the steep times, tea-to-water ratios, and temperatures to discover the flavors you enjoy the most.

> Here's a delightful tip for storing some of your favorite cannabis flowers: Jasmine pearls of any kind will make your cannabis flowers taste even more tantalizing if you keep a few of them in the same jar with your cannabis flowers!

Fresh Market Tea Tasting

One of the most impressive and elegant ways to serve cannabis tea is also the most simple to prepare. The Fresh Market Tea Tasting uses fresh produce, herbs, and flowers paired with high-grade teas and clear cannabis oil concentrates or whole cannabis flowers, depending on the final flavor profile that you seek. This is a Gong Fu style tea service, with just a few modifications to enhance the flavors of the fresh fruits and herbs used in this recipe. This can be steeped multiple times and makes multiple servings.

Select the Flavors:

Try some of my favorite fresh tea combinations or design your own. This recipe chart is your starting guide for a few good tea tastings.

TEA	FRUIT	HERB	FLOWER	ROOT
Sencha	pineapple	lemon grass		
silver needle	blackberry		rose petals	
golden monkey	apple			ginger
oolong	apricot		carnation petals	
Ceylon black	lemon or citron slices		orange blossoms	
Irish breakfast	wild elderberry	lavender		
gunpowder	orange slices (peel removed)		saffron	

Preparation and Service:

1. In a teapot, start with your fresh fruit, steeping in a little hot water while you prepare everything else. In a second teapot, prepare your tea and any dried or fresh herbs for the first rinsing steep to awaken your tea and herbs. You'll be preparing 6 to 8 teaspoons (or about 8 grams) of tea, plus any herbs you would like to add and 6 to 8 ounces (or 200 to 240 milliliters) of water, and steeping at around 200°F (or 93°C) multiple times for 5 to 20 seconds.

2. Measure the Cannabis Infusion Oil into the dropper you will be using to add drops to each serving of tea and set aside.

3. Allow the fresh fruit you have chosen to steep for at least 1 minute in a little hot water. Perform the first steep of your tea and herbs to rinse and awaken them, fill your cups and pitcher to warm them, and then discard this into the basin or over your tea pet on the Gong Fu tray.

4. Pour the fruit and the warm water it has been steeping in into the pot with the tea and herbs, fill the pot with hot water, and perform the second steep for 5 to 30 seconds, depending on the type of tea you have selected. Pour into your pitcher, and then into the cups. Add a drop or two of the Cannabis Infusion Oil to each cup and serve.

5. Repeat step four as many times as you would like by increasing the steep time for a few seconds for each sequential steep. For these infusions, the fruit will already be prepared to release more flavor so you will steep it along with the tea and herbs until everything has steeped as many times as possible to extract all of the flavors.

Tabletop Cannabis Infusion for Beverage and Broth

This is a favorite go-to method of preparing cannabis-infused Western-style teas, herbal tisanes, broths, and dessert beverages at home. Many of the beverage and broth recipes in this book can use this type of cannabis infusion—and I recommend it, as the end result is an infusion that is very light and complementary. It does produce a slightly cloudy liquid, so you'll only want to use it with beverage and broth when clarity is not an issue. This infusion method requires borosilicate glass teaware, which you may already have or you can purchase for a moderate price. The set depicted here is approximately 27 ounces (or 800 milliliters) and can serve six people.

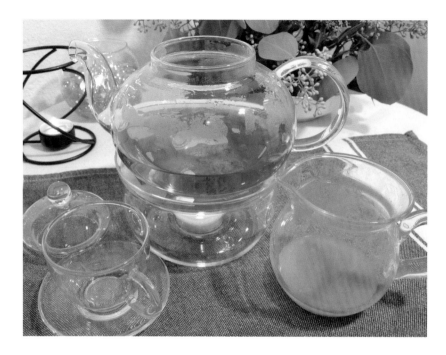

Your borosilicate tea set will include a glass warming dish that operates with a small tea light candle. You may use any tea light candle, but keep in mind that beeswax burns longer and at a higher temperature than most other wax. There may be times where you prefer a little more heat when working with your tea set, so having a few beeswax tea lights around may be useful for you as it has been for me.

Tabletop Cannabis Infusion Ingredients

You'll work with two key ingredients for this infusion recipe: powdered sunflower lecithin and Senegal acacia gum powder. Liquid sunflower lecithin will not work for this infusion recipe; no oil is required. The cannabinoids will infuse and emulsify into the infusion liquid that you create

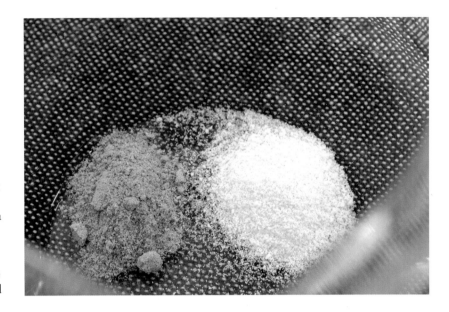

Tools:
1 borosilicate tea set that includes a warming dish for use with a tea light candle
1 small borosilicate glass bowl or brewing pitcher to prepare the cannabis infusion and decarboxylation
1 small whisk
Cups, bowls, or other serviceware for serving the beverage or broth

Ingredients:
Powdered sunflower lecithin
Powdered high-grade Senegal acacia gum*
Cold water
Cannabis concentrate or flowers

*I prefer Heather's Tummy Fiber in the individual serving packets for the freshest acacia gum and best results.

with your tea set, which will be added to the beverage or broth you have prepared and warmed in the glass teapot that comes with your tea set. You'll want to select cannabis concentrate or flower, depending on the flavor profile you desire in your final tea or tisane.

Tabletop Cannabis Infusion for Beverage and Broth Method

Cannabis Infusion Liquid Formulation:

The ratios of powdered sunflower lecithin, Senegal acacia gum, and cold water that you prepare will depend on the form and amount of cannabis you're using. The more lecithin you need to use to emulsify the cannabinoids, the cloudier a beverage or broth may appear at the final service. A premium grade of powdered sunflower lecithin should have a neutral flavor that does not override the flavors in the tea or tisane. Flavor is important here. Selecting the best ingredients is essential.

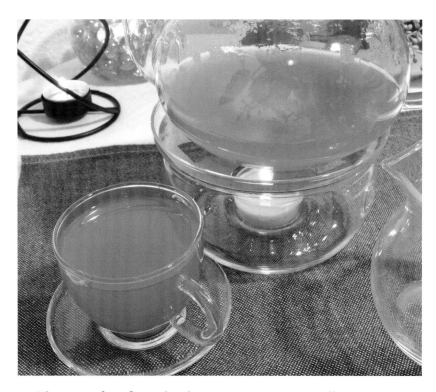

The ratio of sunflower lecithin to acacia gum is usually one-part sun-flower lecithin and two-parts acacia gum. This base formulation works to infuse up to 12 ounces (360 milliliters) of beverage or broth, typically two or four servings, depending on the cup size. My typical recipe to serve two people 6 ounces (180 milliliters) of tea each is ⅛ teaspoon (0.31 grams) of sunflower lecithin and ¼ teaspoon (0.63 grams) of Senegal acacia gum dissolved in 2 tablespoons (30 milliliters) of cold water. Cannabis concentrate containing 40 milligrams of THC is then added to this liquid and processed as instructed here for two servings of tea with 20 milligrams of THC per serving. If you are processing flowers, use 1 tablespoon (15 milliliters) more of water in this formula:

⅛ teaspoon (0.31 grams) powdered sunflower lecithin

¼ teaspoon (0.63 grams) powdered Senegal acacia gum

3 tablespoons (45 milliliters) cold water

Your desired amount of cannabis concentrate or flower

Preparation and Service:

1. In the small borosilicate bowl or pitcher, add the powdered sunflower lecithin, Senegal acacia gum, and the cold water. Thoroughly whisk until dissolved. Light the tea candle and place it inside the tea warmer for your tea pot. Put the grate on the tea warmer and set your infusion bowl or pitcher on top of it.

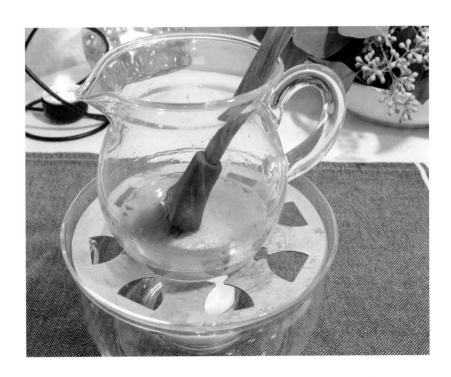

2. While the liquid in your infusion pot is beginning to warm, grind the cannabis flower or add the cannabis concentrate based on the milligram calculations you learned earlier in this chapter. Whisk these into the liquid in your glass bowl or pitcher thoroughly.

3. Allow the cannabinoids to infuse and decarboxylate in the liquid for at least 30 minutes for the best results, adding a little more water to maintain the original level of the liquid, if necessary. Whisk several times during this process. Incidentally, I sometimes hurry this up by 15 minutes using a beeswax tea light when I do not want to wait and have always been pleased with the results. Your bowl or pitcher will process the infusion liquid beautifully with just the heat of the tea light candle.

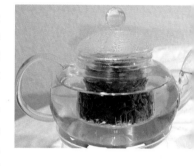

4. Prepare your beverage or broth and set this on the tea warmer as you remove the bowl or pitcher that contains the now ready Tabletop Cannabis Infusion. You may also prepare your broth in a tureen for service and add the infusion into the tureen instead of using the teapot and tea warmer.

5. After 2 to 5 minutes, depending on the appropriate preparation or steeping time for the beverage or broth that you have selected, remove the glass tea infuser from the teapot and set aside if you have prepared tea or herbs. Add the contents of the glass bowl or pitcher containing the Tabletop Cannabis Infusion Liquid to the fresh beverage or broth in your pot or tureen and whisk thoroughly. If you have used ground cannabis flowers, strain out the plant material before pouring the infusion into the teapot.

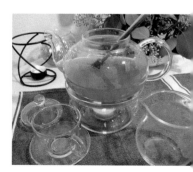

6. You may now pour individual servings of the beverage or broth. Any beverage or broth left in the pot should remain on top of the tea warmer and be thoroughly whisked again before serving more. If you are serving broth from a tureen instead, whisk it again before serving more.

The Art of Cannabis Tea

Tea culture and tasting are refined culinary arts that have been written about and practiced for thousands of years. Masters of the art of selecting and preparing tea have trained for decades as tea sommeliers. Visiting a shop or sommelier with a generous selection of teas to sample is the first step in making a memorable pot of tea, especially if you are serving guests. Tea is a lot like wine—and that's why I think the best tea is the tea you enjoy the most. Appreciating tea, like appreciating wine, does not have to be unapproachable or unattainable in your kitchen. Cannabis tea service can be anything from cozy to formal and everything in between. A humble afternoon cannabis tea among friends can be exuberant, enlightening, and visually stunning when served with the entourage of herbal terpenes in the chapters that follow.

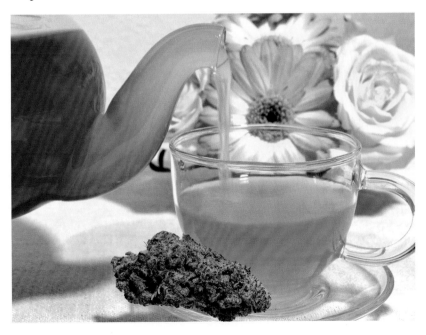

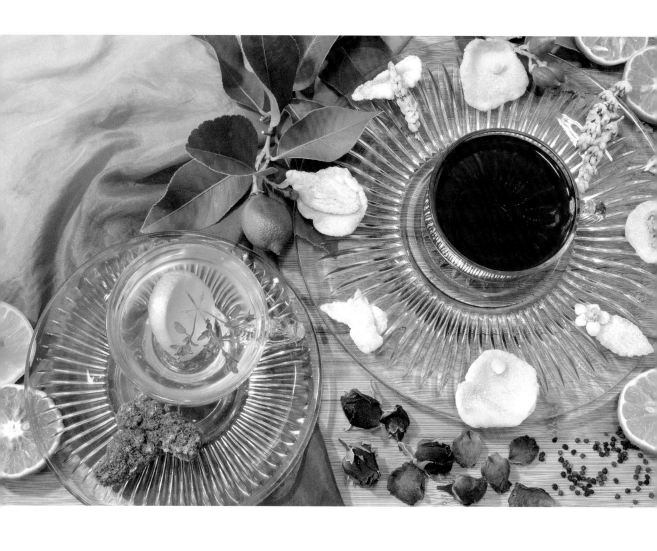

CHAPTER ONE

THE ENTOURAGE TEA

A Symphony for the Mind, Body, and Spirit

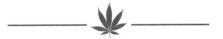

What is Entourage Tea?

Entourage Tea is a method of serving the cannabis-infused tea, tisane, or broth of your choice with delicate candied or spiced fresh herbs, flowers, and fruits to facilitate the joyful reunion of terpenes with cannabinoids in the cannabis tea experience. The method for these candied and spiced terpene entourages is a simple recipe. The final product is shelf-stable and can be stored in a tightly sealed container for up to three months to retain the beautiful color, shape, and terpene content of whatever flowers, fruit, or herbs you choose to candy or spice with this method.

In this chapter, you'll learn the simple steps to make, cure, and enjoy sweet and savory terpene-rich herbs, flowers, and fruits to accompany cannabis-infused tea, tisane, and broth. I call this Turn on, Taste it, and Drop In because that's how these delicate terpene entourages are best enjoyed in the recipes that follow. I think Dr. Leary would be delighted!

Welcome Back What You've Been Missing

Modern cannabis cuisine is quite different from the brownies you used to sneak with your friends in the college dorms. The pungent and grassy

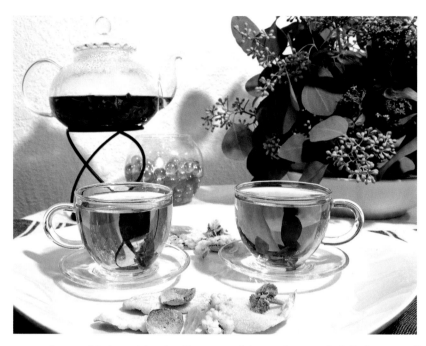

taste of cannabis in cuisine is often something to be avoided. Infusions of precisely measured cannabinoids that have been stripped of their terpenes allow a chef to create their own flavor and fragrance palette that reflects our modern consumption preferences.

But at what cost?

Modern cannabis cuisine often eliminates the typical fragrance and flavor of cannabis, and thus, much of the terpene entourage. But the truth is that even cooking with cannabis the old-school, whole-plant way also entails a great deal of loss in terms of terpene profile.

Terpenes are extremely fragile—and if you've ever experimented with essential oils like lavender, lemon, or rose, you know how quickly they dissipate. This also happens with cannabis flowers as they naturally cure.

Cannabis flowers are always losing terpenes as the flowers age, and once cannabis is reduced to hash or resins, more terpenes are lost.

But why does this matter?

It matters because the entire cannabis experience from top to bottom is predicated on something that has been identified by science and medical professionals like Dr. Sanjay Gupta as the Entourage Effect. Cannabinoids work best with an entourage of terpenes. And welcoming back our favorite terpenes is a simple task because we can find these same terpenes in many familiar fruits, flowers, and herbs.

I believe cannabis cuisine is a more satisfying and healing experience when we welcome back some of the more desirable members of the entourage—like limonene (also found in citrus), linalool (also found in lavender), pinene (also found in rosemary flowers), etc.

For the purposes of creating lovely bouquets of terpenes to infuse into tea, tisane, or broth, the focus here is on the most common terpenes found in cannabis and easily-sourced flowers, herbs, fruits, and spices. There are dozens of terpenes in cannabis, and you'll find it's worth it to check out some of the scientific resources available online to discover more about them. This chart lists five of the most common terpenes found in cannabis and their presence in other edible plants. I've described the experience with the effects of each terpene listed here based on my experiences as well as my guests'.

Tea, tisane, and broth are the perfect culinary canvases to explore cannabis infusions married with some of their naturally occurring terpenes again using fruits, flowers, spices, and herbs. If you've had difficulty finding a positive experience with cannabis cuisine, or if you want to try a different way of experiencing edible cannabinoids, customize your cannabis beverage or broth experience with a terpene entourage to dial in a flavor, mood, and setting that is right for you or your special occasion. I am confident

Common Cannabis Terpenes and their Fruit, Flower, Herb, and Spice Correspondences

TERPENE	FRUITS, FLOWERS, HERBS, SPICES	ENTOURAGE ENHANCEMENT
Limonene	lemon, orange, citron, herbs like lemon balm or lemon thyme	energizing, uplifting, anti-depressant, pain relieving
Linalool	lavender, some basil varieties	sleep, anti-anxiety, quiet focus
Pinene	rosemary, pine needles, juniper berries	memory enhancing, anti-depressant, invigorating
Myrcene	mango, hops, lemongrass	muscle relaxation, sleep, stress relief
Caryophyllene	black pepper, clove, carnation	anti-anxiety, pain management, stimulating/relaxing

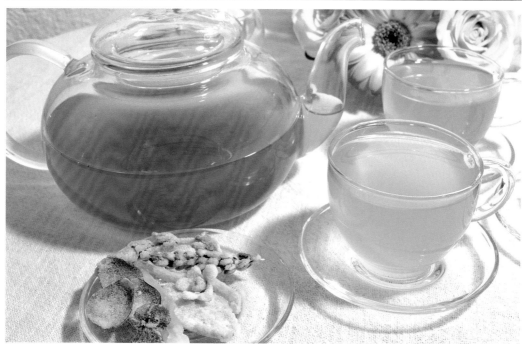

this method of preparing and serving cannabis tea, tisane, and broth will be a satisfying one.

Transforming Herbs, Spices, Flowers, and Fruits into a Terpene Entourage

You'll be using both fresh and dried varieties of many different herbs, spices, flowers, and fruits to create terpene entourages for your tea service. The recipe chart included here has many interesting terpene combinations, but you are really only limited by your imagination!

The Process

Terpene entourages are created using a very high grade of Senegal acacia gum in a fragrant and mildly acidic liquid (citric or acetic), which is then dipped in a caster sugar, caster xylitol, or powdered herbs or spices. This is left to dry on a drying plate or rack on parchment paper and is typically dry within two to three days, depending on environmental humidity. The process of painting or dipping the herb, spice, flower, or fruit in the acacia gum liquid

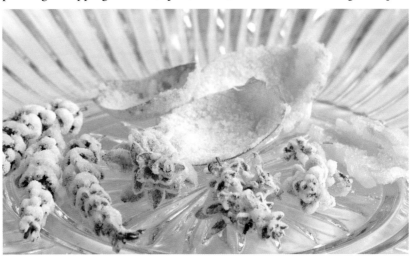

and coating with caster sugar, xylitol, or powdered spices is very astringent and draws moisture out of them quickly while retaining the shape and color.

Bakers are no doubt familiar with candied rose petals and flowers—a specialty item used to dress up cakes and other baked goods. Typically, these are dipped in or painted with egg whites and coated in caster sugar before being left to dry. While this method may be acceptable for traditional baked goods, it's not the best, and it's not free of major allergens (eggs). It also does not have the astringent or preservation advantages of working with a very high grade of Senegal acacia gum. Preparing fresh herbs and flowers as terpene entourages using Senegal acacia gum captures their terpenes and allows for terpene layering via hydrosols like rosewater, fragrant tea, or herbal waters. And unlike egg white preparations, these are shelf-stable in a closed jar for many months while retaining their natural color and shape. These are created for cannabis tea, tisane, or broth, but you can also use them for traditional baked goods—they are very fragrant, beautiful, and completely edible.

The Ingredients and Tools

- *Fresh herbs* like basil flowers and tops, rosemary flowers, lavender flower spikes, mint leaves or flowers, lemon thyme, tender lemongrass.
- *Fresh flowers* like rose petals and small cored buds, citrus blossoms, blackberry blossoms, cherry blossoms, chamomile flowers, violets, carnations.
- *Fresh fruits and spices* like shaved citrus peels, shaved ginger root, shaved turmeric root.
- *Dried spices* like black peppercorns, clove buds, cardamom seeds.
- *Hydrosols, distilled water, teas, and herbal waters* like rosewater, orange blossom water, mint water, green tea, lemon balm water infusion.

- *Caster sugar (baker's sugar), caster xylitol, and powdered spices* like cinnamon, smoked paprika, curry, or powdered herbs. Do not use regular sugar or xylitol—the grains are too heavy and will weigh down your delicate herbs and flowers. Xylitol or sugar can be milled into a caster-sized grain using a blender or coffee grinder.
- *Senegal acacia gum* is also known as gum arabic. The grade that we use to create our terpene entourage is a very high grade Senegal acacia gum, *Acacia Senegal*—and this distinction is important because not all acacia gum or gum arabic is the fine grade of *Acacia senegal.* You will want to purchase this as a powder to create the liquid that will be used to dip or paint your herbs, fruits, spices, and flowers. In my experience, the highest grade of this acacia gum comes as a powder for use as dietary fiber. Heather's Tummy Fiber is a reliable and authentic *Acacia senegal* brand that is powdered and works well in the recipes in this book.

  The properties of a high-quality Senegal acacia gum are essential to making and enjoying these terpene entourages with tea, tisane, or broth. This fiber, unlike other fiber or cheaper fiber, will not gel or change the texture of the hot liquids when the herbal entourage is steeped or dropped into them. The acacia gum will also aid in firming the emulsion of oils and cannabinoids in the tea, tisane, or broth they are paired with, as explained in the introduction chapter of this book.
- *Lemon or lime juice, citric acid, acetic acid (distilled vinegar)* improves flavor and color preservation and creates a slightly acidic environment that is less friendly to unwanted microbiology.
- *Assorted soft paint brushes and tweezers for manipulating the delicate herbs* are essential for getting just the right amount of acacia liquid on your herbs, flowers, fruits, and spices. I use a fan brush and a fine detail brush for even coverage.

- *A drying rack or plate covered with parchment paper and cheesecloth to cover the terpene entourages* while they air dry. Alternatively, you can dry them in a food dehydrator at room temperature or a bit warmer with the fan on high.

The Tea and Terpene Entourage Experience: Making, Pairing, Tasting

Making terpene entourages involves a simple part-for-part recipe to coat and preserve the shape, essential oils (terpenes), and color of whatever herb, flower, fruit, or spice you select that is then dusted or buried in caster sugar, caster xylitol, or a powdered spice before being air-dried.

There are many variations for this coating—you are really only limited by your imagination! The recipe formula itself looks like this:

1 part Senegal acacia gum powder +
1½ parts clear liquid (distilled water, culinary hydrosols like rosewater, green tea, etc.) +
½ part acidic liquid (lemon juice, lime juice, distilled vinegar, etc.)

OR

1 part Senegal acacia gum powder +
2 parts clear liquid (distilled water, culinary hydrosols like rosewater, green tea, etc.) +
⅛ part citric acid crystals

I prefer fresh lemon juice for most of my terpene entourages, but you may want to experiment with these variations to create your own layers of flavor and fragrance.

HERB, FLOWER, OR FRUIT	CLEAR AND FRAGRANT LIQUIDS	ACIDIFIER	SWEETENER	PRIMARY TERPENE EXPERIENCE
lemon peel	rosewater	lemon juice	caster sugar or caster xylitol	limonene, geraniol
black peppercorn	rosewater	lemon juice	caster sugar or caster xylitol	caryophyllene, damascenone
rose petal / cored rosebud	rosewater	lemon juice	caster sugar or caster xylitol	geraniol, damascenone
lavender spike	green tea	lemon juice	caster sugar or caster xylitol	linalool, pinene
blackberry blossom	orange flower water	lemon juice	caster sugar or caster xylitol	nerol, geraniol
Greek basil flowers	rosewater	lime juice	caster sugar or caster xylitol	myrcene, linalool
blood orange peel	rosewater	lime juice	caster sugar or caster xylitol	limonene, myrcene
lemon thyme	distilled water	lemon juice	caster sugar or caster xylitol	limonene, myrcene
rosemary flowers	distilled water	lemon juice	caster sugar or caster xylitol	pinene, camphor

Here's a standard recipe that I use frequently for my terpene entourages:

Instructions:

Thoroughly mix all ingredients until smooth with a light syrup-like texture. Use within a day. This small amount will cover several bunches of herbs and flowers! Quite often, even this small recipe will have leftover liquid when I am finished—a small amount goes a long way.

The Terpene Entourage Recipe Chart

This recipe chart has formulations that have been tried and tested in my own kitchen and on my tea-time guests for the best results and feedback. These are suggestions, not rules, so get creative with what you have locally and in your own kitchen!

You will want to begin with very clean and fresh herbs. If you're working with green herbs and flowers or flower petals, note that these are quite delicate and will wilt fast if they are not floated in a bowl of water while you are working. One of my favorite tricks for really infusing fresh herbs and flowers with even more fragrance is to float them in a bowl of mint, rose, or orange flower water while I am working.

It's important to remember that the fresh herbs, flowers, and fruits you work with should have enough of their mass exposed to air to dry properly. For example, lemon peels should be prepared not by using the whole peel, pith and all, but rather using a potato peeler or zester to shave off thin peels from the outside of the rind.

The Terpene Entourage Preparation Method:

1. With your tweezers, carefully pick up the herb or flower by the stem or other small edge and use your paintbrush to coat the surfaces. You may also dip into the liquid

1 tablespoon (5 grams) powdered Senegal acacia gum

1½ tablespoons (22 milliliters) culinary rosewater

½ tablespoon (8 milliliters) lemon juice

Alternatively, if you would like to use citric acid instead of lemon, lime, or vinegar:

1 tablespoon (5 grams) powdered Senegal acacia gum

2 tablespoons (30 milliliters) culinary rosewater (or any fragrant water or hydrosol)

⅛ teaspoon (0.31 gram) citric acid

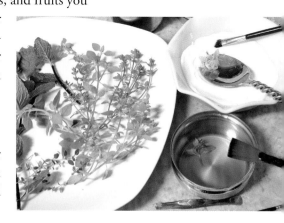

and then manipulate with the tweezers to tap off the excess. You do not want a thick coating that is too saturated, but you do want to cover the surfaces completely. If you're working with a flower or other herb that has complex surface areas that can cup or hold too much of the liquid (like the inside of a blossom), be sure to tap this out gently so that the crevices are not filled with liquid. This will oversaturate the coating of sugar, xylitol, or powdered spice that is applied before drying.

2. If you have just coated a leaf, lemon peel, or flower petal, you may now bury this in the bowl you have set up with sugar, xylitol, or powdered spice. Using your tweezers, carefully pick it up out of the bowl and gently tap before putting in the final drying area. If you're working with a blossom or other flower with a more complex surface area, instead of burying, you'll want to carefully dust it with one of the dry ingredients. To do so, continue holding it with your tweezers and use a small spoon or dry brush to dust the sugar, xylitol, or spice over the surfaces to cover them without weighing down the delicate areas.

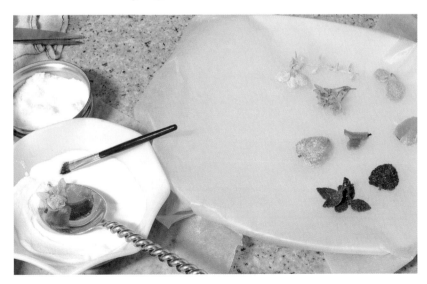

3. In humid environments, you may want to dry these on the high fan and no or very low heat setting of your dehydrator. In most environments, these will dry completely in the open air within a day or two. Some, like lemon peels, may require an extra day or two.

4. Your final dried terpene entourages will look almost ceramic after drying—and if you have used sugar or xylitol, they will sparkle! Store these in a tightly closed jar only after they are fully dry. Adding a humidity pack or other humidity control pack to the jar will help to extend their shelf-life.

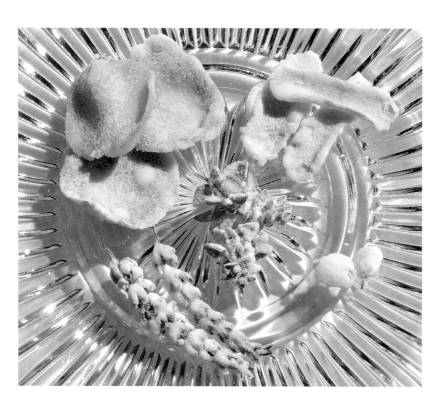

Enjoy! The Entourage Tea Recipes

In the introduction to this book, you've learned how to make emulsifiable cannabis infusion oil that works well in clear liquids like Gong Fu tea service as well as a cannabis infusion sans oil that is very light and works well will many other beverages and broths. You'll be using the infusion recipes from the introduction in these tea recipes, which are accompanied by terpene entourages.

Teas are brewed with very hot to boiling water. Many tea connoisseurs may be curious as to why this is. The answer is that the cups of tea, tisane, or broth need to steam sufficiently to raise the bouquet of essential oils (terpenes) from the terpene entourages that have been dropped into the cup up and into the nose—this is the first wave of the terpene entourage experience. When you serve into cups or bowls from a teapot or pan, you will want sufficient heat to produce some rising steam from the cups for a few seconds while terpene entourages are selected, tasted, and then dropped into the cups. To that end, the tea selections in this chapter are made with a higher temperature brewing. Adjust steeping times to control astringency or bitterness.

The second wave of the terpene entourage experience is the infusion of the essential oils into the tea itself. You will taste these as you sip. In your cup, the terpene entourages will marry their coatings with the hot liquid and take shape in the cup as though they were fresh blooms and herbs! The acacia gum acts to quickly preserve and draw out moisture from the herb or flower as it dries and then rehydrates beautifully in your cup. The acacia gum coating the entourages acts as an additional emulsifier for the essential oils and cannabinoids in the hot liquid. Swish or stir your terpene entourage in the cup as you enjoy the beverage.

The terpene entourages also make luscious, sweet, and spicy nibbles. There's nothing quite like biting into a candied lemon peel or rose petal while sipping tea—delicious, with an enchanting flavor that will expand all over your palate.

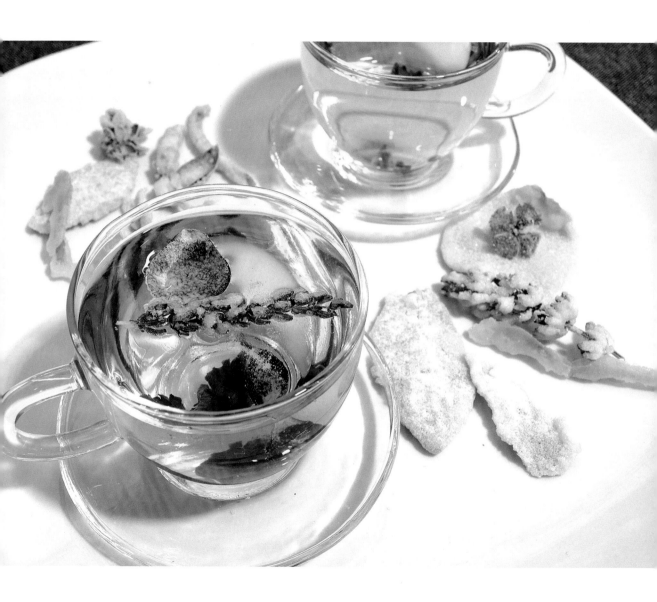

Vanilla Milk Oolong Cannabis Tea with Lavender Spike or Ginger Entourage

Measured doses of the
   Cannabis Infusion Oil
   (Page 11) in a dropper
6–8 teaspoons (about 8
   grams) milk oolong tea
1 thumbnail-sized piece of
   vanilla bean, chopped
8 ounces (240 milliliters)
   water per steeping
Lavender spike or ginger
   slice terpene entourage

Milk oolong, otherwise known as Jin Xuan, is a very special tea grown in the high mountains of Taiwan and is notable for its unique flavor profile of milk, butter, and peaches. Care is required when purchasing milk oolong—only the highest grade will do, as many of the lower grades have dairy flavorings infused into the tea to compensate for their lack of flavor. Authentic milk oolong contains no added flavorings and has never touched a dairy product of any kind to achieve its creamy flavor.

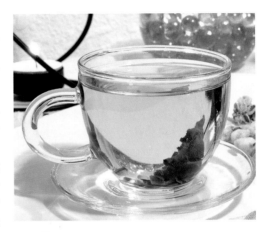

For this recipe, you will need a thumbnail-sized piece of vanilla bean to brew with the tea. Lavender spike entourages are my favorite to serve with this tea, but another favorite is ginger root. You can serve one or both! Makes many servings when prepared Gong Fu-style, which is the style of preparation recommended for this type of tea.

Preparation:

1. Prepare the Cannabis Infusion Oil in your dropper and set aside. Begin tea preparation of milk oolong by rinsing in a first steep, and discarding the tea in the basin or over your tea pet. Add the vanilla bean pieces and tea to the glass basket of your tea pot with a small amount of water in the bottom (but not touching the glass tea basket) as shown here. Heat

water for brewing while the tea leaves and vanilla are warming. Arrange the selected terpene entourages on a separate plate or on the teacup plate next to the cup.

2. Pour the hot water over the tea, and perform a 5 to 10 second steep. Then remove the filter basket from the teapot.

3. Serve the tea in slightly larger cups than are normally used to serve Gong Fu style to accommodate the terpene entourage in the cup. Add 1 to 3 drops of the Cannabis Infusion Oil to the cups, and serve each time you steep. You and your guests may now swirl the oil in the cups and drop the entourages directly into the hot tea to release the terpenes and sweeten the tea.

4. Continue to re-steep the tea in the filter basket until the leaves are finished. You should be able to get multiple infusions before the leaves are spent.

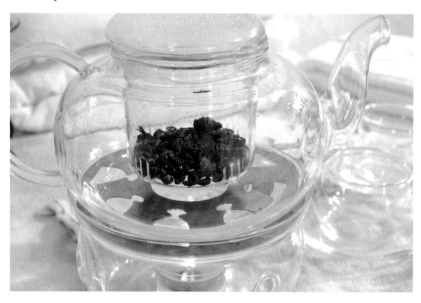

Moroccan Green and Saffron Cannabis Tea with Pink Mint Entourage

2 servings of the cannabis infusion of your choice (Cannabis Infusion Oil, page 11, or the Tabletop Cannabis Infusion, page 33)

2 teaspoons (5 grams) Moroccan-style or Gunpowder green tea

5 or more saffron threads

12–16 ounces (360–480 milliliters) water (2 servings)

Pink mint terpene entourage, for garnish and to sweeten

Moroccan style green teas are robust with flavor as well as caffeine—and even have a similar "crema" to espresso coffee due to the method of preparation and the richness of this tea. Moroccan tea is poured from a foot or more above the teacup to create this crema on top of the tea before drinking. A few threads of saffron completes the flavor of this kind of tea, making it more floral and soft. Served with this Moroccan-style cannabis tea is an entourage of pink mints created using mint leaves and caster sugar that has had a drop or two of pokeberry juice worked into the crystals by stirring. I explain more about pokeberry in the second chapter of this book (see page 66), but you can use a drop or two of any pink or red vegetable

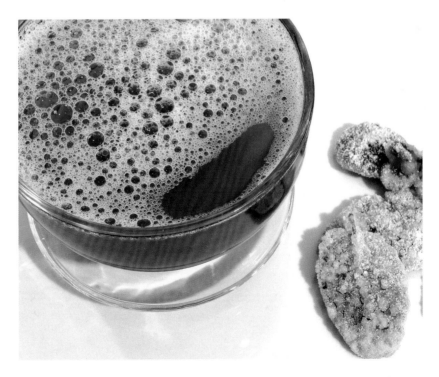

dye to give these candied mint leaves the pink color that looks so pretty when served with this tea. Makes 2 or more servings.

Preparation:
1. Select one of the cannabis infusion methods and prepare a pot of tea. Infuse the tea after brewing for 1 minute or more and removing the filter basket.
2. Prepare the pink mint entourage for this tea using the method described in this chapter (page 50). Arrange the pink mint entourage on the plates next to the cups, one or two for each cup of tea served.
3. Whisk vigorously and then pour the tea into the cups high above the cup to create the desired crema, and serve immediately.

Raspberry Black Pearl Cannabis Tea with Rose Petal Entourage

Black pearl is an oxidized but not fermented rolled tea that is rich and smooth. It has the body necessary to support both bold and delicate spices and herbs. Raspberry black pearl served with rose petal terpene entourage is one of my very best tea recipes. For this tea, I use freeze-dried raspberries for the most concentrated flavor, but you may use fresh berries if you have those on hand. I typically prepare this tea in the longer Western-steeping style, and it makes 2 or more servings.

2 servings of the cannabis infusion of your choice (Cannabis Infusion Oil, page 11, or the Tabletop Cannabis Infusion, page 33)

3–5 large black dragon pearls

5–7 freeze-dried raspberries

12–16 ounces (360–480 milliliters) water (2 servings)

Rose petal terpene entourage, for garnish and to sweeten

Preparation:
1. Select the cannabis infusion method you would like to use from the introductory chapter and prepare it. Prepare the basket in your teapot with berries on the bottom of the filter basket and the tea on top for the best flavor after steeping. You should be able to get at least two infusions from this tea when it is done Western-style.
2. Steep the tea for at least 2 minutes or more. Arrange the rose petal entourage on the plates next to the cups, one or two for each cup of tea served. Remove the filter basket of tea and add the cannabis infusion you have selected, whisk, and serve.

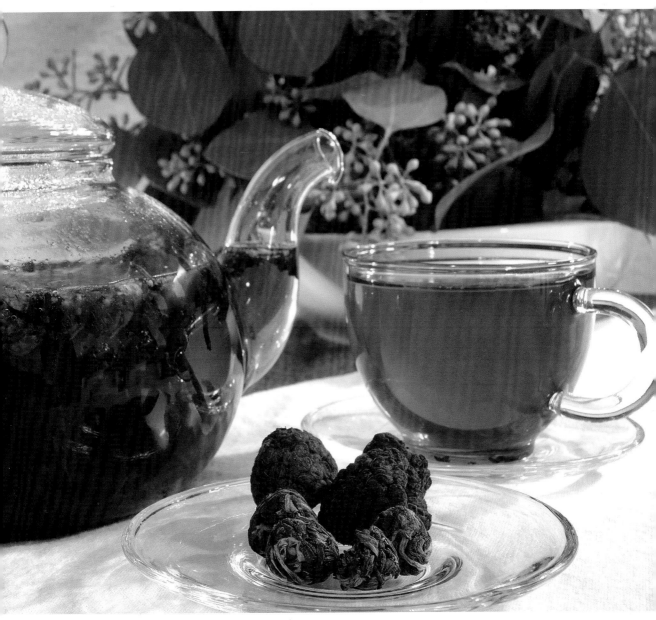

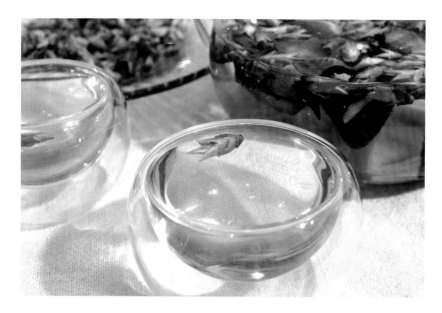

Yabao Fresh Market Cannabis Tea with Entourage

Yabao is one of the most interesting teas out there—and one of the few pu'erh teas sun-dried straight from the bush with no other processing or fermentation. It's difficult to find but not as expensive as you would expect for such a rare tea product. Yabao looks and tastes like no other tea. It's hard to describe—floral, dry, piney, and you may taste some spice in there from time to time. It's a delicate little bud harvested in the early spring from wild tea bushes. Yabao looks like white tea, but the liquor of this tea is even lighter than most white teas. The crisp, light color and dry flavor can host any flower, herb, or fruit you want to pair with it! I think that is what makes it really special and one of my favorite teas for infusing with cannabis.

Yabao has no upward or downward limit on steeping time or water temperature; it never gets bitter or astringent. It is the most "mistake-proof" tea you will ever prepare and is sure to impress even the most discriminating

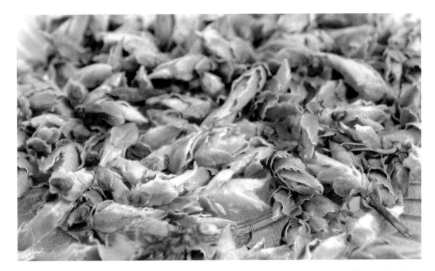

of palettes. Yabao is an excellent tea for terpene entourages of any kind—sweet or spicy. It can be prepared Gong Fu or Western-style, so experiment with what you like.

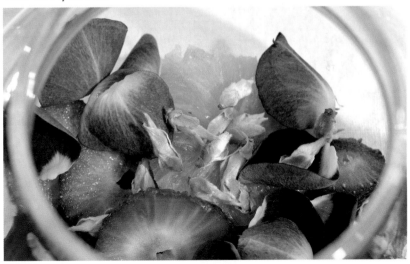

Try some roses, hibiscus flowers, lavender flowers, apples, or berries, and see if you don't agree that this tea is perfect with fresh market flavors. You'll want to pair this kind of infusion with a very clean cannabis extract with little or no flavor of its own for the best results. However, a cannabis flower with a very unique fragrance can play quite nicely with yabao, so don't rule out whole-flower infusions with this tea. Makes 2 or more servings.

Create the Pot:

In the filter basket of your tea pot, loosely layer 8 grams or more of the tea with your choice of cut fruit, berries, herbs, and fragrant flowers—one or more of these. Or enjoy yabao tea simply on its own and serve with complementary terpene entourage.

Preparation and Service:

1. Select either the Cannabis Infusion Oil method (page 11) or the Tabletop Cannabis Infusion method (page 33). The instructions here reflect more of a Western-style tea preparation, so if you choose to prepare this Gong Fu, select the Cannabis Infusion Oil, as the Tabletop Cannabis Infusion does not work well with Gong Fu preparation.

2. Bring 12 to 16 ounces (360–480 milliliters) of water (2 servings) to a boil, and pour over the filter basket in the pot. Steep at least 3 minutes or even more before removing the filter basket and whisking in your cannabis infusion selection. After service, you may put the filter basket back into the teapot and steep in fresh water again for as long as you like or even all day! Yabao tea can remain in the pot indefinitely; it does not get bitter and has the interesting feature of changing flavor profiles as it continues to steep. Serve with terpene entourage.

3. You may continue to serve tea from the pot into the previous cups with the cannabis infusion. Feel free to infuse with cannabis again, or just enjoy the tea by itself.

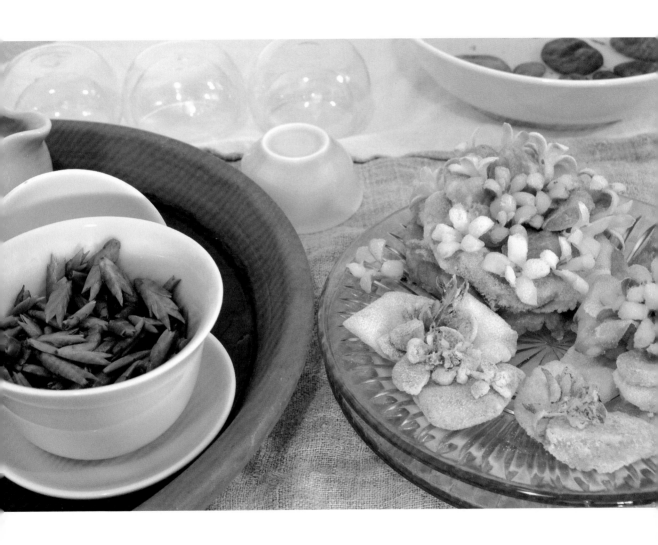

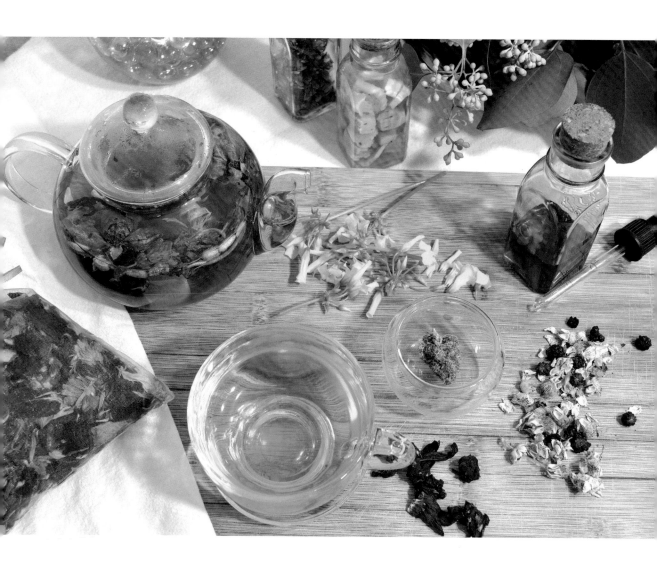

CHAPTER TWO

CANNABIS HERBAL TISANES AND ENTOURAGE FOR WELLNESS

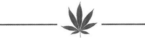

Cannabis is a plant teacher that has helped me to connect with other plant teachers in a meaningful way—and this is very much what this chapter is about. Many of the tisane recipes in this chapter have been inspired by the plants themselves found on my many gathering adventures in the wilds of California. It is my hope that you will be delighted and enlightened by them and will connect with them in the way I have while enjoying all of the herbal wellness they have to offer.

Let's Take a Walk on the Wild Side

I don't make my love of wildcrafting a secret. Some of the most fascinating and delicious herbs and fruits I have encountered have been on a stretch of wild trails, fields, and woodlands on a few hundred acres owned by a good friend of mine. One of my favorite pastimes is the wildcrafting of invasive plant species, of which there are many here in California.

I will admit that I live a little dangerously while gathering in the wild. Sometimes I'll taste things as they present themselves to me even if I am not quite sure what they are. I feel a deep, spiritual connection to this gathering activity, and I allow the plants teach me as I go along. I'm also a very experienced home herbalist with more than twenty years of collecting and consuming many kinds of plants, but you don't need my years of experience to get out there and let the plant teachers speak to you.

The best advice I can give to those seeking new plant teachers and reconnecting with their primal gathering instincts is to educate yourself on the basics of what grows wild in your locality as well as any potential harmful effects of the plants that you forage. When in doubt, just leave it alone—good advice, even if I don't always follow it.

Pokeberry: The Healer

Pokeberry, poke, cancer root, otherwise known as *Phytolacca americana,* is an invasive plant species in California native to the Appalachian and southern states. It has become naturalized or invasive in almost every state—and yes, it even grows in Europe now, as well. Poke is considered an herbal medicine, a toxic plant, as well as a food in the southern states—the young green shoots are boiled three times and fried to make a springtime dish in the south called poke sallet. As the stems and leaves grow, they become inedible, which is why they are gathered as they are emerging from the ground only in the spring when the toxicity is very low.

Poke is a mild to moderately toxic plant, which, depending on what sources you read, may be described as very dangerous. I personally feel this is alarmist and not as rational as official sources, like CalFlora, in classifying it only as mildly toxic. It's certainly not anything like hemlock. The dried root can be purchased from reputable herbal suppliers online who consider it safe for adults to use with some caveats. Many people consider the constituents of this plant to be quite healing when judiciously used.

I've known about poke for many years. When I was a child, my grandfather, who grew up in the shadow of the Appalachian Mountains, used

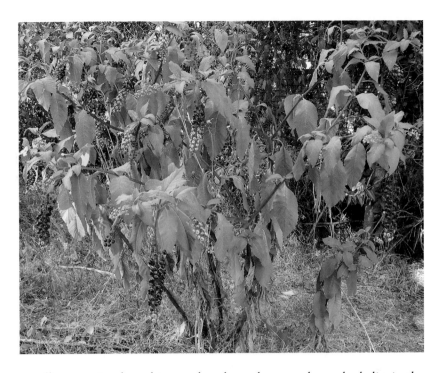

to tell me stories about his grandmother, who was a home herbalist in the late nineteenth and early twentieth century in their Ohio farming community—a community with little or no access to doctors. Back then, what the doctors had to offer in terms of health care was sometimes a lot more dangerous than what the grandmothers in the community were suggesting and using! Nineteenth-century medicine was no joke.

My great-great grandmother, like many of the herbalist grandmothers in that place and time, had a specialty she was called upon to share with the community when people fell ill from life-threatening diseases like cancer. That specialty was her knowledge of working with the poke plant. My grandfather recounted many stories to me of his grandmother's poke root poultices and other preparations with the power to draw tumors out of the body.

While on one of my many foraging adventures in the wilds of California, I was taken by surprise when this magnificent plant teacher with a deep connection to my familial roots introduced itself to me on a disturbed trail—plump, shining berries and all. I knew immediately what this was and initially felt awe as well as a healthy fear of the secrets it held. "It's poisonous. I can't possibly understand the safe ways to work with this plant because this knowledge has been lost in my family," I thought to myself. I paid my respects and kept my distance for a while. But I kept hearing it call to me each time I would walk that trail—and one day that resulted in me bringing home a bag of the berries to experiment with in my own kitchen.

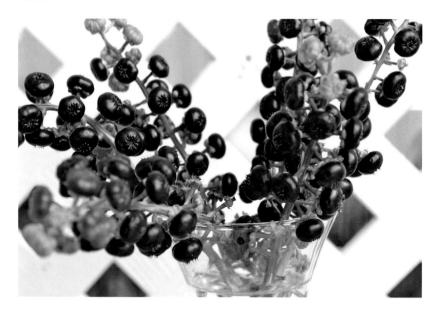

After some time spent with the 1905 edition of the *King's American Dispensatory*, which contains a plethora of information about many of the uses of the poke plant during that period of time that the doctors, pharmacists, and home herbalists relied on, I settled on trying to express the juice of the pokeberry. Specifically, I was interested in the use of this juice for its anti-inflammatory medicinal purposes in a tisane, as a natural and brilliant fuchsia coloring agent for some of my terpene entourages, and to create show-stopping pink sugar. The pokeberry tastes green or grassy, so they aren't included in recipes based on their flavor. The juice from just one or two berries makes anything you put it in quite lovely with a brilliant pink that really pops with color! The pokeberry recipes in this book represent some of the work I have done with this plant.

If you are an adult, it's between you and your doctor to decide which herbs are best for you. Poke contains some chemistry that may not be compatible with your current medications or your unique health situation. That said, the juice of the berries, minus the unbroken seeds, is the safest part of this plant for an herbalist or chef to experiment with, save for the tender young shoots that emerge in the spring. I take the juice from these berries almost daily in my cannabis tisanes. I think the juice has very effective anti-inflammatory properties especially when paired with cannabis and a tasty anti-inflammatory spice like ginger root.

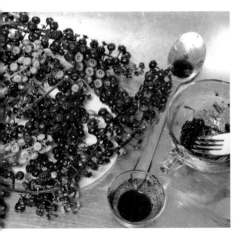

Juicing the Pokeberry

This is a delicate process that should be done carefully by hand. There are a dozen or so black seeds in each berry and all of them are toxic. Crushing, chewing, or blending them in your recipe in any way has been described as dangerous by many sources and should be avoided. The fresh berries are very plump and full of juice. Lightly mashing them and allowing them to sit for a couple hours and then squeezing the juice out of them through cheesecloth produces excellent results. You can freeze the juice in tiny cube sizes and pop them into a cannabis tea or herbal tisane.

Sun-Drying the Pokeberry

These can be dried in the hot summer sun when they reach full maturity. I use a ceramic plate and turn the side plucked from the stem facing upward. In the dry, California summer environment, these berries dry like little raisins in three days. I cover them with a single layer of cheesecloth.

To work with these, you will need to discard any of the berries that go off-color, producing green or brown liquid when re-hydrated. You will need to re-hydrate the berries and remove the seeds before brewing with your teas or tisanes. Soak two or three sun-dried berries in 2 tablespoons of hot water from the tap and allow them to re-hydrate. This should take half an hour. After they're soft, gently mash them to expel all the seeds and then remove them from the liquid. Brew your tisane or tea with the pokeberry liquid, including the skins, and then filter your tea or tisane as you would normally, and serve.

Fresh Ginger and Pokeberry Canna-Tisane

This is a fast and fresh tisane that is not only gorgeous in the cup, but really delivers the wonderful flavor of pure ginger. You can easily pair this with sweet terpene entourages like lemon or citron peel. Use this recipe as a guide to make as many servings as you would like. This recipe makes 1 or 2 servings.

1–2 servings of the cannabis infusion of your choice (Cannabis Infusion Oil page 11, or the Tabletop Cannabis Infusion page 33)
1 large thumb ginger per serving, sliced
1 pokeberry per serving
6–8 ounces (180–240) milliliters water

Preparation:

1. Prepare your cannabis infusion selection. Place the ginger and pokeberry in the teapot, pour boiling water over them, and allow them to steep for 5 minutes over a tea light or on low heat before straining.
2. Strain and then add your cannabis infusion selection, whisk, and serve with terpene entourage, if desired.

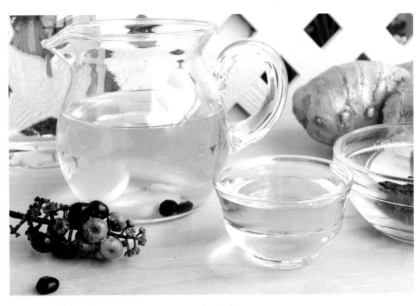

The Anti–Inflammatory Wonder Tisane

1–2 servings of the cannabis infusion of your choice (Cannabis Infusion Oil page 11, or the Tabletop Cannabis Infusion page 33)
1 large thumb ginger per serving, sliced
1 pokeberry per serving
3 black peppercorns per serving
1 thumb-sized turmeric root, chopped
6–8 ounces (180–240 milliliters) water

Similar to the previous tisane, which featured the singular flavor of ginger to pair with terpene entourage, this tisane features both ginger and pokeberry with the addition of two more spices to increase the soothing and pain-relieving effects that you will surely experience as you enjoy one or more servings of this colorful tisane. Use this recipe as a guide to make as many servings as you would like. This recipe makes 1 or 2 servings.

Preparation:

1. Prepare your cannabis infusion selection. Place the ginger, peppercorn, turmeric, and pokeberry in the teapot, pour boiling water over them, and allow them to steep for 5 minutes over a tea light or on low heat before straining.
2. Strain and add your cannabis infusion selection, whisk, and serve with lemon peel or rose terpene entourage to sweeten.

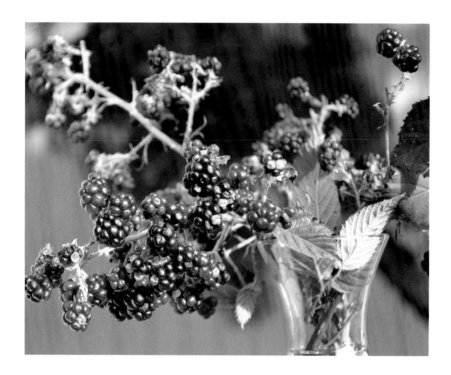

Himalayan Blackberry

Most of the United States and countries in temperate climates, like Europe, have this invasive blackberry species, *Rubus armeniacus*—but it is especially invasive on the west coast. In California, you can find it everywhere. It's a little dangerous, too! If you're going to brave the brambles to forage, wear thick shoes, clothing, and gloves because the thorns are absolutely vicious and will have no mercy for you! The leaf, flower, and fruit have impressive medicinal and culinary features, making this blackberry a must-have in your herbal kitchen—and worth the fearsome trip into the brambles.

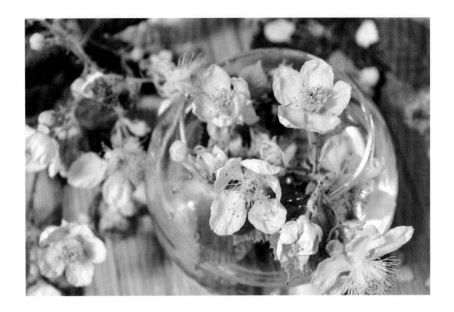

You can find blackberry leaf tisane in your local natural foods store, but I have found this wild species to be much more flavorful, as the tannins can be modified through a curing process to create a very smooth tisane that has the floral and tea-like flavors of teas like oolong tea. The blackberry leaf tastes so much like tea that you can use this as a caffeine-free tisane whenever you want the taste of real tea. Blackberry leaf—whether fresh, dried, or cured—has many facets of flavor like tea leaves, with fresher and greener dried leaves being more tannin and astringent and cured leaves being mellower.

Drying Blackberry Leaves

I prefer sun-drying for almost all herbs because it's fast and efficient. Sun-drying has some sterilization properties that give it a distinct advantage over electric dehydration, namely mold and yeast inhibition. If you live in an especially humid environment, you may want to try a combination of sun-drying and electric dehydration when drying blackberry leaves or any other herb, fruit, or vegetable for the best results. If you choose this method, start by sun-drying for a few hours or a day and then finish in the electric dehydrator.

As soon as you pick blackberry leaves, they can be washed and dried; they do not need to be cured (oxidized) unless you desire that flavor. Try them both ways with cannabis tisane and select the one you like the best. I think the most flavorful blackberry leaves are the new leaves that emerge in the spring and have a lovely fruity and floral flavor, but you can use any blackberry leaf to create a delicious and caffeine-free tisane.

Curing Blackberry Leaves

This is essentially a twenty-four-hour oxidation process that will bleed out a lot of the tart tannins from the blackberry leaves for a smooth and delicious tea-like tisane. It does not involve fermentation. This process works best with older blackberry leaves. Very young leaves that have just emerged from the cane can be wilted in the sun with similar results.

Gather and wash the blackberry leaves. I like the younger leaves the best, but I have completed this curing process with a mix of old and new leaves with really great results. After washing, take a paring knife and scrape the thorny spine off the back of the older leaves and discard.

1. Using a rolling pin or similar kitchen tool, roll and bruise the leaves significantly until they are limp and every part has been bruised.
2. Using a clean damp cloth, wrap the leaves and keep the cloth damp for 24 hours. The leaves will bleed a significant amount of their tannins and may now be a dark green to brownish-black color. A good cure will also result in a slightly floral or fresh fragrance from the bruised leaves as they release tannin.

3. Remove the leaves from the damp cloth and dry them immediately in the sun or in a dehydrator on a very high fan setting and high heat to avoid any formation of mold. I prefer sundried leaves, and it only takes about a day in the hot sun and a dry environment to completely dry them.
4. Store the dried blackberry leaves in a closed container and use the same amount as you would when brewing a regular cup of tea.

Wild Himalayan Blackberry Leaf Canna-Tisane Blend

Because the blackberry leaf is so versatile, you can blend this with many other flavors—the ones here with mint and elderberry flowers are one of my favorite to blend with blackberry leaves for tisane. However, any spice or herb that is tasty with regular tea will also pair nicely with this. And blackberry leaf has some interesting medicinal properties that work well

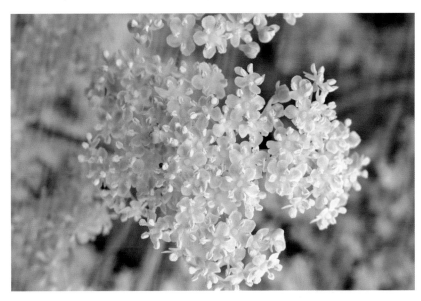

with cannabis to soothe upset stomachs. This recipe blends blackberry leaf with other soothing herbs for a well-rounded, caffeine-free herbal tisane that is delicious any time of the day or night. Makes 2 servings, or a little more.

Preparation:

1. Prepare your cannabis infusion selection. Brew the blackberry leaf, mint leaf, and elderberry flowers as you would a typical tea: 2 minutes of steeping time or fewer for the best floral flavors.
2. Strain the herbs and add your cannabis infusion selection, whisk, and serve with honey or terpene entourage to sweeten if you desire.

Blackberry Blossom and Blood Orange Canna-Tisane

Fresh California blood oranges plucked from the tree are among my favorite things during citrus season when these are so abundant. Fresh blood

2 servings of the cannabis infusion of your choice (Cannabis Infusion Oil page 11, or the Tabletop Cannabis Infusion page 33)
1 tablespoon (about 2 grams) dried or dry-cured blackberry leaf (include some dried blackberry flowers for more flavor!)
½ teaspoon (0.25 grams) dried mint leaf
1 teaspoon (.50 grams) dried elderberry flowers
12–16 ounces (360–480 milliliters) water
Honey or terpene entourages, as desired

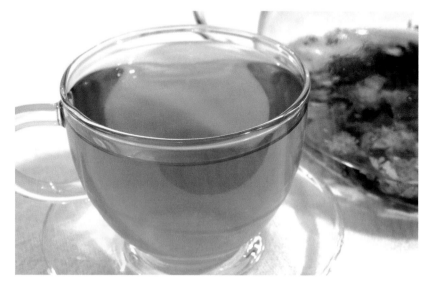

2 servings of the cannabis infusion of your choice (Cannabis Infusion Oil page 11, or the Tabletop Cannabis Infusion page 33)

1 tablespoon (3 grams) dried blackberry blossoms and a few dried blackberries

1 teaspoon (0.50 grams) blackberry leaves

1–2 slices whole blood orange, peels removed

12–16 ounces (360–480 milliliters) water

Honey or terpene entourage, to sweeten

oranges from the tree have a yum factor that is awesome in just about anything, including fresh tisane. Blackberry blossoms have that same tea-like flavor as blackberry leaves but with a hint of floral. Tisane with blackberry blossom and fresh blood orange slices is perfect for a caffeine-free breakfast. Enjoy this with a biscuit or scone or just by itself.

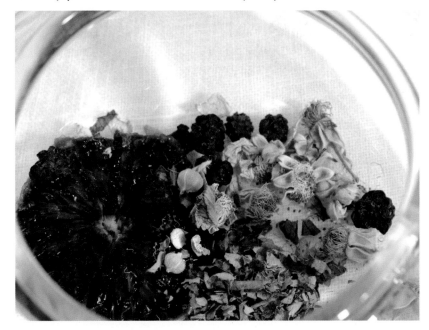

Try my method of warming a pot of honey to serve with this tisane! Makes 2 servings, or a little more.

Preparation:

1. Prepare your cannabis infusion selection. Brew the blackberry blossoms, blackberries, blackberry leaves, and orange slices more than you typically do with tea or tisane: steep 3 minutes or more.

2. Strain the herbs and add your cannabis infusion selection, whisk, and serve with honey or terpene entourage to sweeten if you desire.

The Wild Olive

All the wild olive trees we have on the west coast of California were at one time cultivated olive trees. What makes them "wild" now is that they are invasive—and when they establish themselves in the wild, their fruit changes, typically becoming smaller and drier. I often dry-salt cure these wild olives over a number of weeks and have found them to be highly concentrated with a rich olive flavor that cannot be found in any supermarket.

But, did you know the olive tree bears a medicinal leaf that has been used for centuries as a delicious tisane for whatever ails you? Olive leaf

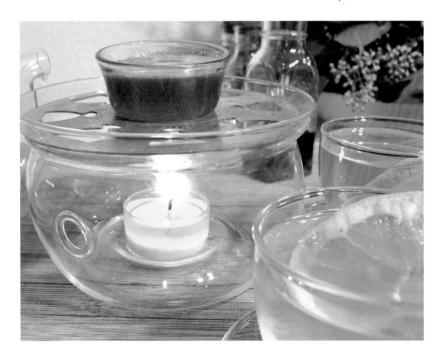

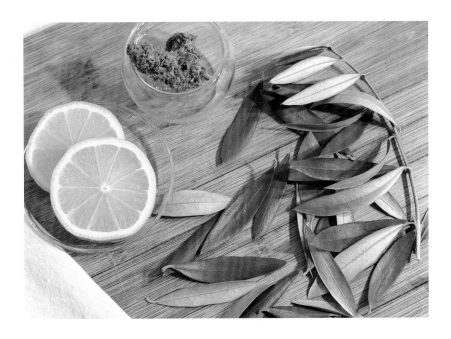

tisane is similar to green tea with a slight bitterness from the oleuropein contained within the leaves. Olive leaf tisane can be as delicious as it is healing if you have acquired a taste for it. If you want to try an energizing tisane that is a real fatigue-fighter with some noteworthy anti-inflammatory effects, and caffeine-free, olive leaf is perfect.

My cannabis and olive leaf tisane has been prepared using sun-dried olive leaves that have been exposed to the sun, outside, for several days to one week on a ceramic plate covered with one layer of cheesecloth.

Olive Leaf, Mint, and Citron Canna–Cleanse Tisane

This very cleansing and refreshing olive leaf blend creates a lively Mediterranean tisane that is energizing and bright. The tisane will brew faster and a bit stronger if the leaves are broken, but you can enjoy the

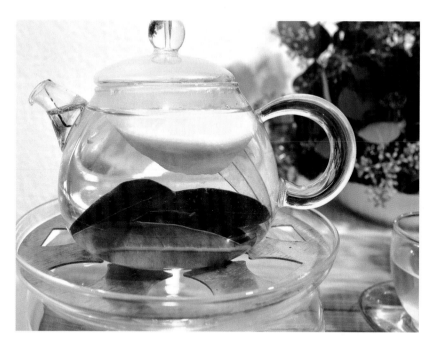

2 servings of the cannabis infusion of your choice (Cannabis Infusion Oil page 11, or the Tabletop Cannabis Infusion page 33)

2 teaspoons (2 grams) dried olive leaves, coarsely crushed or whole

1 teaspoon (0.50 grams) dried mint leaves

1 teaspoon (1 gram) citron peel, chopped, or 1 slice of lemon

12–16 ounces (360–480 milliliters) water

lighter flavor and body of the whole leaf tisane, if you prefer that. I like to infuse this with a micro dose of cannabinoids from sativa strains to rescue me from fatigue and clear all of the brain fog! Makes 2 servings.

Preparation:
1. Prepare your cannabis infusion selection. Steep the olive leaf, mint leaf, and citron peel for at least 3 minutes before infusing with cannabis.
2. Strain the herbs and add your cannabis infusion selection, whisk, and serve.

Western Blue Elderberry

All along the west coast of the United States and into Mexico is a species of elderberry native to this area. This is known as the blue elderberry,

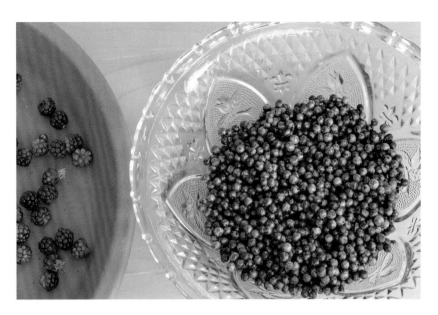

or *Sambucus nigra* ssp. *cerulea*, due to the blue color of the berries that are different from the commercial and wild European black elderberry, *Sambucus nigra*, which most people are familiar with.

Gathering the blue elderberry in the wild will certainly reflect in the flavor of these berries. Here in the very dry environment of California, they have a very concentrated flavor that can be best described as blackberry, raisin, blueberry, plum, and a hint of orange blossom all at once. These are a beautiful fruit for tea, tisane, and baking, but they also have the wonderful medicinal properties that the European black elderberry has. Enjoy this vital berry only after heating or drying in the sun, as they are slightly toxic when raw.

Breathe Easy, Speak Easy Canna–Tisane

This is a fantastic seasonal tisane for sore throats, colds, and allergies. I like to infuse this with CBD-rich cannabis concentrate or flower for a more restful sleep and clear sinuses. I harvest eucalyptus leaves (the blue gum variety) locally from the wild here in northern California as well as western white pine needles, also foraged locally. Makes 2 servings.

Preparation:

1. Prepare your cannabis infusion method (Cannabis Infusion Oil on page 11, or the Tabletop Cannabis Infusion on page 33). Boil the water and then pour over the lemon, mint leaf, eucalyptus leaf, pine needles, and elderberries, and allow them to steep for at least 5 minutes over your tea light warmer before straining and then infusing the tisane with cannabis. Whisk vigorously.
2. Serve with honey or ginger terpene entourage to sweeten, if desired.

Sassafras

Another plant that gets a bad rap from the government is sassafras, or *Sassafras albidum*. Selling the bark for tisane became quasi-illegal in the sixties and seventies in the United States because the FDA posted warnings about sassafras tisane being carcinogenic.[4] Later, with the rise of MDMA or "ecstasy," sassafras oil came under severe scrutiny and regulation by the DEA. Safrole, one of the essential oils in sassafras, is a precursor for making MDMA.

I was introduced to sassafras tisane by my grandfather when I was a child in elementary school. For many decades, I have pined for the flavor of this tisane but only recently have been able to find the bark for sale on Amazon and other retail sites. It was very exciting to try this tisane again after so many years.

2 servings of the cannabis infusion of your choice (Cannabis Infusion Oil page 11, or the Tabletop Cannabis Infusion page 33)

2 slices whole lemons, peels removed

1 teaspoon (0.50 grams) dried mint leaves

3 or 4 crushed dried eucalyptus leaves

2 teaspoons (1 gram) white pine needles, chopped

1 teaspoon dried elderberries (2 grams) or 1 tablespoon (3 grams) fresh elderberries

12–16 ounces (360–480 milliliters) water

Honey to sweeten or serve with ginger peel terpene entourage

---

4   CFR—Code of Federal Regulations Title 21
      http://www.accessdata.fda.gov/scripts/cdrh/cfdocs/cfcfr/CFRSearch.cfm?fr=
      189.180

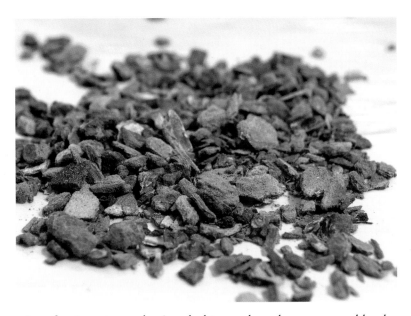

Sassafras is native to the Appalachian and southern states and has been used for hundreds of years as a delicious tisane served hot or cold by the people of these regions. Many old-timers still harvest the bark for tisane even though the government would prefer they didn't. As an adult, it's up to you to decide if you think the government has once again overstated the negative effects and overstepped their bounds regarding a plant.

I treat sassafras with respect and use it sparingly in the spring and fall—no more than once or twice a month. I think this is a wonderful tisane with a lot of vitality and a unique flavor that cannot be duplicated. And sassafras really is a gem in the cup with its rich, garnet-like color, layers of flavor, and fragrance of spice and floral that has a distinct Victorian-era feeling, as this was the main ingredient of the root beers of that period. Victorians relied on sassafras tisane as an uplifting tonic in the spring that chased away the sluggishness after a long winter and again when the light started to fade quickly in the fall.

Sassafras Canna-Tisane

I believe that my Sassafras Canna-Tisane will brighten your soul and awaken your mind as it has done for me as a seasonal tisane. Enjoy this with floral terpene entourage like citrus blossom, blackberry blossom, jasmine blossom, lavender, or rose petal as a drop-in to enhance its refreshing qualities. Makes 2 servings, or a little more.

2 servings of the cannabis infusion of your choice (Cannabis Infusion Oil page 11, or the Tabletop Cannabis Infusion page 33)

3 teaspoons (5 grams) dried sassafras bark

12–16 ounces (360–480 milliliters) water

Sorghum molasses to sweeten, or serve with floral terpene entourage

Preparation:

1. Prepare your cannabis infusion method (Cannabis Infusion Oil on page 11, or the Tabletop Cannabis Infusion on page 33). Boil the water

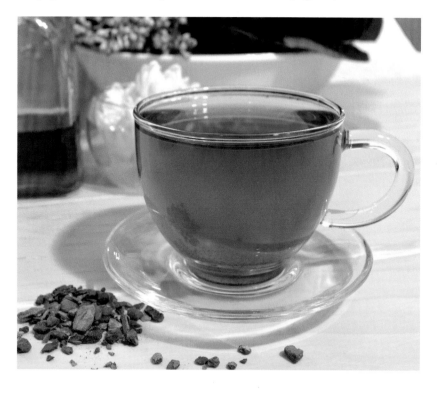

and pour it over the sassafras bark in your teapot filter basket. Steep it in hot water for at least 10 minutes over your tea light warmer before straining and then infusing with cannabis. Whisk vigorously.

2. Serve with sorghum molasses, or floral terpene entourage, to sweeten if you desire.

Canna–Tisane: My Favorite Blends

Jah's Good Hibiscus Spice Canna–Tisane

2 servings of the cannabis infusion of your choice (Cannabis Infusion Oil page 11, or the Tabletop Cannabis Infusion page 33)
3 or more whole dried hibiscus flowers, broken into pieces
1 whole cinnamon stick or pieces
4 whole allspice
2 or 3 slices of fresh ginger
12–16 ounces (360–480 milliliters) water
Honey, or serve with floral terpene entourage

I am always in awe of the beauty and flavor of island cuisine, but especially Ital cuisine from Jamaica. Hibiscus tisane is a favorite of the island folk and one that really deserves a spot on your tea table from time to time. Makes 2 servings, or a little more.

Preparation:

1. Prepare your cannabis infusion method (Cannabis Infusion Oil on page 11, or the Tabletop Cannabis Infusion on page 33). Boil the water and pour this over the hibiscus and spices. Steep for at least 5 to 10 minutes over your tea light warmer before straining and then infusing with cannabis. Whisk vigorously.
2. Serve with honey, or floral terpene entourage, to sweeten if you desire.

Foggy Beach Herbal CBD Tisane for Restful Sleep

CBD oils are very popular in the states where cannabis has been legalized for a variety of reasons, ranging from very serious illness to simply needing a more restful sleep. This tisane is inspired by all of the foggy afternoons I

2 servings of the cannabis infusion of your choice made with flower or oil rich in CBD, (Cannabis Infusion Oil page 11, or the Tabletop Cannabis Infusion page 33)

3 teaspoons (2 grams) chamomile flowers

5 or more dried or fresh strawberries (wild is preferred)

1 teaspoon (0.50 grams) lemongrass

12–16 ounces (360–480 milliliters) water

Lavender honey or lavender spike terpene entourage, to sweeten

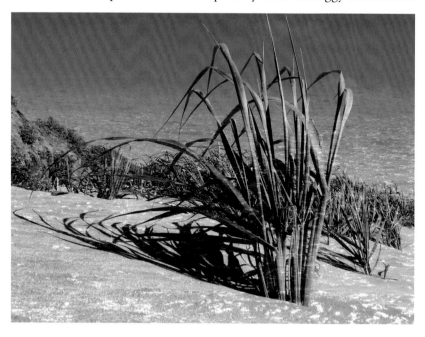

spent in Pacifica, California, and the wild strawberry I discovered growing there and around Half Moon Bay. However, you may use any strawberry fruit that you have on hand. Makes 2 servings.

2 servings of the cannabis infusion of your choice (Cannabis Infusion Oil page 11, or the Tabletop Cannabis Infusion page 33)

1 teaspoon (0.50 grams) blackberry flowers (substitute cured blackberry leaves if you don't have any flowers)

5 strands saffron

2 teaspoons (1 gram) rose petals and buds

1 teaspoon (0.50 grams) jasmine flowers or orange blossoms or both combined or ½ teaspoon (2.5 milliliters) orange flower water

½ teaspoon (0.25 grams) fennel flowers

1 teaspoon (0.50 grams) lavender flowers

5 dried hibiscus flower petals

½ teaspoon (0.25 grams) lemon thyme or melissa (lemon balm)

12–16 ounces (360–480 milliliters) water

Honey or citrus terpene entourage, to sweeten

Preparation:

1. Prepare your cannabis infusion method (Cannabis Infusion Oil on page 11, or the Tabletop Cannabis Infusion on page 33). Boil the water and then steep all the herbs and strawberries for at least 3 minutes over your tea light warmer before straining and then infusing with cannabis. If you are using orange flower water, add this after your tisane has finished steeping.

2. Strain the herbs and add your cannabis infusion selection, whisk, and serve with lavender honey, or lavender spike terpene entourage, to sweeten if you desire.

Many Flowers Cannabis Enlightenment Tisane

Zhourat is the Arabic name for a many flowers caffeine-free tisane, which is an essential in the tea culture of the Middle East and especially Syria. You may purchase it in almost any Arabic grocer stateside, but blending your own is satisfying, as you can blend any number of flowers and herbs that you have on hand. There are so many ways to make this tisane—you are not limited by the floral blend I suggest here. I do think that blackberry blossoms give this a stable underpinning to hold the rest of the floral flavors in this tisane, though. This is the perfect meditation tisane for yoga time, spiritual meditation, or really any time. Makes 2 servings.

Preparation:

1. Prepare your cannabis infusion method (Cannabis Infusion Oil on page 11, or the Tabletop Cannabis Infusion on page 33). Boil the water and pour it over the flowers, and allow to steep for 2 to 3 minutes. Strain and then add the cannabis infusion. Whisk vigorously.

2. Serve with honey or citrus terpene entourage to sweeten if you desire.

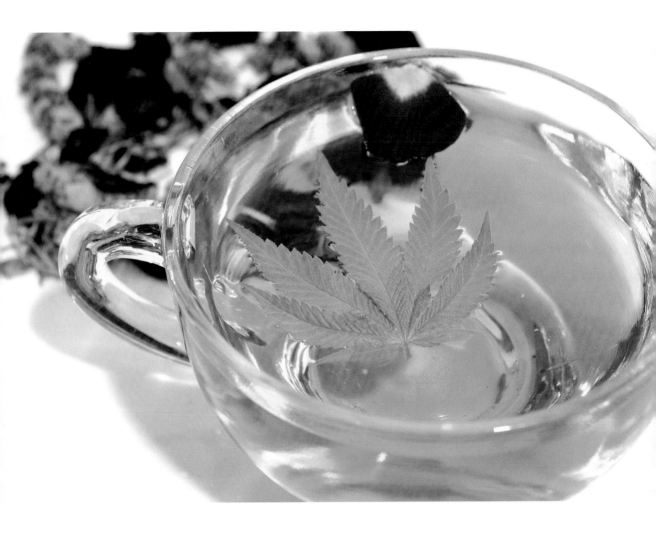

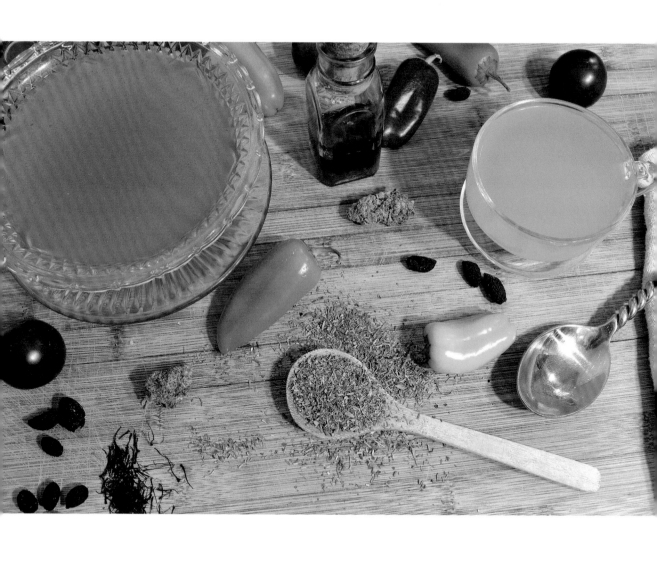

CHAPTER THREE

A SAVORY ENTOURAGE

Satisfying Cannabis Broths

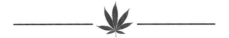

Broth: A Savory Cannabis Infusion

I did not feel that this book of gracious cannabis tea-time recipes would be complete without a chapter filled with my favorite cannabis-infused broth recipes. Both vegetable and bone broths are quite popular these days; they are nutritious, light, and satisfying. Making your own broth is easy, but it will require at least 4 hours (and up to 12 hours of cook time for larger bones on your stove) so save these recipes for your designated cooking day. They may be frozen and reheated for a quick, savory indulgence anytime.

Terpene Entourage for Cannabis Broth

In chapter 1, you were introduced to the terpene entourage. These are herbs, flowers, or fruits coated with a mixture of acacia gum, fragrant culinary water, and an acidic liquid like lemon juice, caster sugar, xylitol, or powdered spices. They capture many of the same essential oil terpenes found in cannabis like limonene, linalool, and pinene, which are also found in many other herbs, flowers, and fruits. These boost the flavor and effectiveness of cannabinoids that have been infused into beverages or broths.

In this chapter, we will select and make terpene entourages to taste and drop into our cannabis-infused broth. Instead of sweet entourage, these herbs, flowers, and fruits are coated with powdered spices. For your convenience, I've included the liquid acacia gum formula from chapter 1 for dipping and painting the fresh herbs, flowers, or fruits before they are coated in powdered spices and dried, along with a spices chart to inspire your own creations.

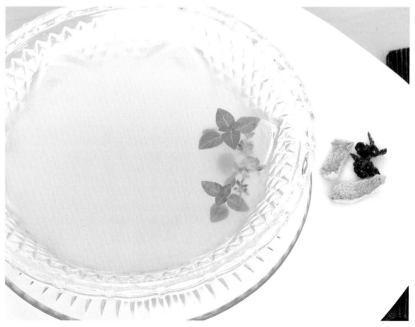

1 part Senegal acacia gum powder +
1½ parts clear liquid (distilled water, culinary hydrosols like rosewater, green tea, etc.) +
½ part acidic liquid (lemon juice, lime juice, distilled vinegar, etc.)

OR

1 part Senegal acacia gum powder +
2 parts clear liquid (distilled water, culinary hydrosols like rosewater, green tea, etc.) +
⅛ part citric acid crystals

HERB, FLOWER, OR FRUIT	CLEAR AND FRAGRANT LIQUIDS	ACIDIFIER	SPICE	PRIMARY TERPENE EXPERIENCE
lemon peel	green tea	lemon juice	powdered ginger	limonene
black peppercorn	tulsi tea	lemon juice	curry powder	caryophyllene
rose petal / cored rosebud	rosewater	lemon juice	powdered sumac	geraniol, damascenone
ginger slice	green tea	lime juice	hot chili powder	linalool, myrcene
rosemary tips or flowers	rosemary tea	lemon juice	powdered white pepper	nerol, pinene
basil tips or flowers	orange flower water	lemon juice	Jamaican jerk spice blend	myrcene, nerol

The Basic Cannabis Broth Recipe

You will be using this basic broth-making recipe with all of the broth recipes in this chapter. It makes 1 quart (about 1 liter) of broth or more depending on what you are using to make the broth and how much water is boiled away. This can be doubled or more if you are making broth to freeze or serve more than four guests 8-ounce (240-milliliter) servings. Broths generally keep well in the refrigerator up to three days for the best flavor. Freeze if you are not going to use it by then.

Preparation:

1. Select and prepare your cannabis infusion and set aside. In a pan on the stove, put all of the vegetables, bones, and seasonings into a stockpot with the water. Bring this to a rolling boil and then turn down to a simmer. You will be simmering this pot at least 4 to 12 hours, depending

4 or more servings of the cannabis infusion of your choice (Cannabis Infusion Oil page 11, or the Tabletop Cannabis Infusion page 33)

2 quarts (2 liters) water (or more)

Vegetables, seasonings, and bones as specified in each individual recipe blend in this chapter

Terpene entourage, as desired

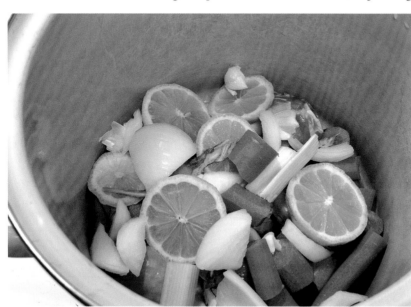

on the ingredients in each of the recipes. Bones make the best broth when they are simmered for at least 8 hours. You may add more water during the boil, if necessary. Stocks will reduce as much as half of the amount of liquid you started with before they become flavorful.

2. During the first hours of simmering uncovered, you will notice the broth produces a foam or "scum" at the top in most bone broths. You will want to continually skim this off until it stops forming during the simmering process. You may then cover it for the remainder of the simmering time (most likely 1 hour) to lock in more flavor. I like to add the fresh herbs I will be using during the last hour of the simmer for more enhanced flavor.

3. You will know when your broth is ready when all the vegetables, most bones, and herbs are mostly mushy, the stock is reduced in volume, and the broth tastes very flavorful. If it is too bland, boil to reduce the amount of water in the stock to concentrate the flavor even more. Remove this from the stove and allow it to cool enough so that you can run it through a standard kitchen strainer.

4. After you have strained all the ingredients from your broth, you will strain the broth again through several layers of cheesecloth into a clean pan. Place the new pan on the stove and heat again before adding the cannabis infusion. If you have been working with bones, allow the stock to cool before reheating so that you can skim the fat from the top before returning it to the stove.

5. Heat the broth until it begins to steam and vigorously whisk in the cannabis infusion you have already selected and set aside. Serve in a tureen, bowls, or cups immediately with terpene entourage, or allow it to cool to room temperature and then refrigerate. Freeze after refrigerating for several hours if you do not intended to use the broth within three days.

6. When reheating this broth, always whisk vigorously to evenly distribute all the cannabinoids.

Cannabis-Infused Broth Recipe Blends

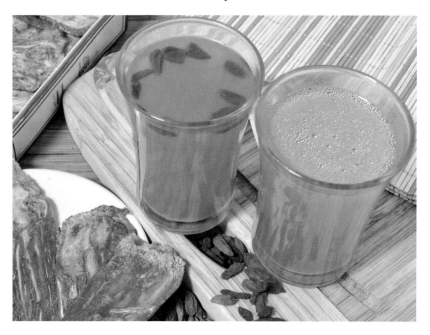

Women's Canna–Tonic Broth

My best broth for whatever feminine complaint is ailing you! PMS? Cramps? Menopause? Ah, yes . . . menopause . . . my favorite! I sure do not enjoy feeling like someone has just lit my head on fire while sitting at my desk. And by golly, that's why I really dig this broth recipe for relieving uncomfortable symptoms like hot flashes and crankiness. Cannabis adds another dimension to this for cooling, pain relief, and mood management. Yeah, you ladies out there know what I'm talking about!

4 or more chicken legs or 1 small chicken carcass
1 or more large slices of Dong Quai root

15 red Chinese dates
2 or 3 medium-sized carrots
2 slices whole lemon
2 or 3 medium-sized cloves of garlic
Sea salt and cracked black pepper, to taste

Follow the instructions for basic cannabis broth on page 94. Serve with goji berries to garnish or ginger citrus terpene entourage.

Elderberry Lemon Thyme Canna–Chicken Broth

The ultimate prescription for colds, flu, and seasonal allergies has always been the quintessential chicken soup or chicken broth. The recipe for this is pretty much the same in every kitchen, but for this seasonal broth to scare away the bugs, we're going to infuse it with the wild blue Western elderberry you learned about in chapter 2 along with whole lemons and fresh thyme. The end result is a delicious chicken broth with the brilliant color and surprising flavor of elderberry.

3–4 chicken legs or 1 small chicken carcass
½ medium onion
3 large cloves garlic
2 or 3 medium-sized carrots
2 stalks celery
1 medium lemon, sliced
1 small bunch (5 stems) thyme
1 teaspoon dried elderberries (2 grams) or 1 tablespoon (3 grams) fresh
    elderberries
½ teaspoon (0.50 grams) white pepper
Sea salt and cracked black pepper, to taste

Follow the instructions for basic cannabis broth on page 94 and make adjustments as necessary.

Lemongrass Ginger Chili Canna-Chicken Broth

This is a lively Thai cuisine–inspired broth with the three essential flavors of this cuisine: lemongrass, ginger, and chili. These create a bright and warm broth perfect for any season of the year. Serve with a terpene entourage made with Jamaican spice blend!

4 chicken legs or 1 small chicken carcass
2 large thumbs ginger, sliced
3 or 4 dried chili pods of your choice (or less, depending on the heat you
   like)
2 large (or 5 small) stalks of fresh lemongrass, chopped
½ small lemon, sliced
2 or 3 medium-sized carrots
1 stalk celery
5 garlic cloves
Sea salt, to taste

Follow the instructions for basic cannabis broth on page 94 and make adjustments as necessary.

Cipollini Onion and Peppercorn Canna-Beef Broth

This is a fantastic herbal onion broth to make with the bones from a cowboy steak or roast. It makes a great starter, as well as a nice dipping broth for the arrowroot breadsticks in chapter 5 (page 141).

1 roast bone or 1 or more cowboy steak bone (bison or venison bones are great, too!)
15 or more cipollini onions or a mix of cipollini and shallots
2 medium cloves garlic
Handful parsley
Handful fresh marjoram
2 teaspoons (3 grams) black peppercorns
Sea salt, to taste

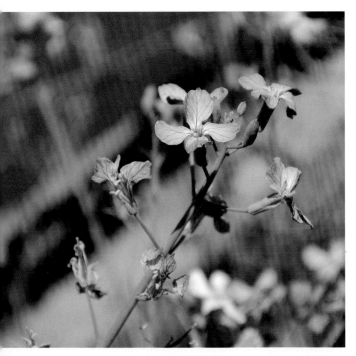

Follow the instructions for basic cannabis broth on page 94 and make adjustments as necessary. Bone broths such as this one typically require 8 to 12 hours of simmer time on the stove for the best flavor. Garnish with wild radish blossoms for a special presentation.

Seven Herb Canna-Vegetable Broth

Herbes of Provence are a popular French seasoning blend for all kinds of recipes. I love making broth with this blend of herbs because the flavors are so exciting, people often ask me what is in it! The secret is seven herbs: marjoram, thyme, rosemary, lavender, summer savory, oregano, and basil. That's my blend, but everyone has their favorite style of making this so go with your heart and taste buds on this one or pick up an already blended version of this seasoning at your local supermarket.

You may select whatever vegetables are in your refrigerator and need to be used right away to make this broth. Some of my favorites are onion, pepper, garlic, celery, carrot, squash, and maybe one medium tomato.

1 tablespoon (or 6 grams) Herbes de Provence
Veggies from the fridge, such as:
    5 large carrots
    3 stalks celery
    2 large sweet peppers
    1 large onion
    1 medium tomato
    1 medium courgette
    1 large garlic clove
Sea salt and cracked pepper, to taste

Follow the instructions for basic cannabis broth on page 94 and make adjustments as necessary.

Sicilian-Style Canna-Vegetable Broth

This is a tomato-based vegetable broth with a few interesting twists. It uses wild, salt-cured olives to add a deep flavor note that is almost "meaty" as well as one of my other favorite ingredients—fennel flowers. It features

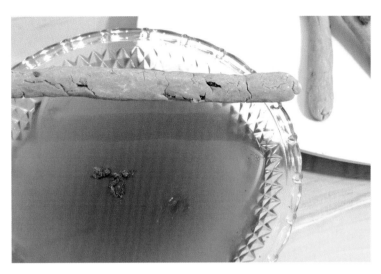

peppers and onions, too. If you can't find fennel pollen or flowers, you can use a cut fennel bulb.

5–10 fresh and very ripe roma tomatoes
1 large bell pepper (orange or red for best broth color)
3 large cloves garlic
2 large carrots
Handful fennel flowers or ½ fennel bulb
1 teaspoon (1 gram) black peppercorns
2 whole dried red-hot chilies
1 small bunch (3–4 stems) fresh marjoram
1 medium onion
5 or more dry, salt-cured black olives
Sea salt, to taste

Follow the instructions for basic cannabis broth on page 94 and make adjustments as necessary.

Curried Canna-Vegetable Broth

This is a very spicy and energizing broth to be enjoyed when you want a great pick-me-up. It features fresh root spices like ginger and turmeric and is meant to be garnished with a garam masala blend. Perfect for afternoon tea time or 4:20 p.m.!

Veggies from the fridge, your choice
3 cloves garlic
1 large thumb ginger, chopped
1 large turmeric root, chopped
1 small bunch cilantro
1 teaspoon (2 grams) cumin
1 whole cut lemon
5 cracked cardamom pods
1 cinnamon stick
10 cloves
2 teaspoons (3 grams) black peppercorns
½ teaspoon (1.5 grams) mustard seeds
½ teaspoon (1 gram) fennel seeds
Sea salt, to taste

Follow the instructions for basic cannabis broth on page 94 and make adjustments as necessary. Note that this recipe is even more awesome if you cut up a small, ripe mango without the skin and cook it in the broth.

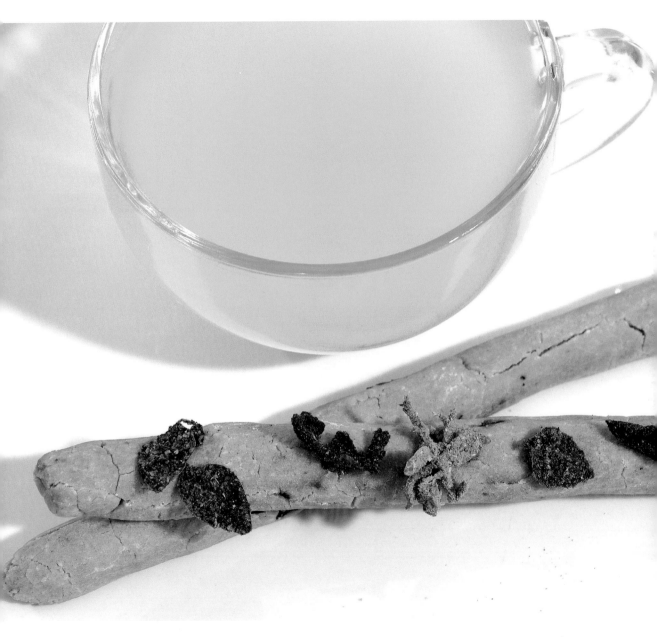

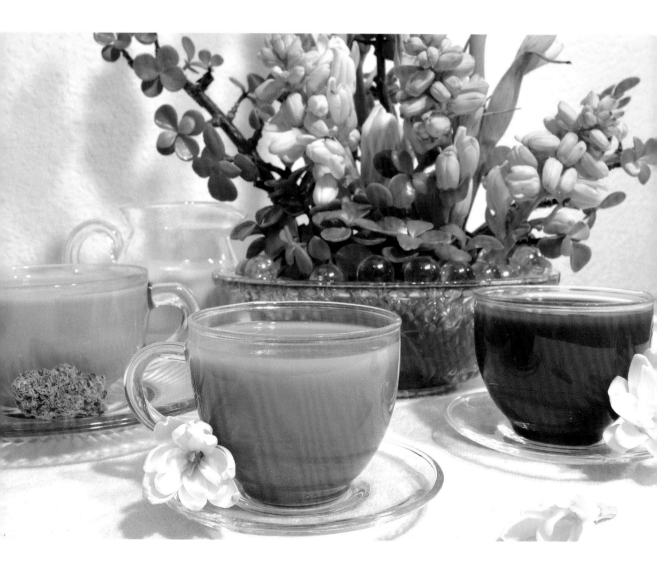

CHAPTER FOUR

BHANG, CHAI, AND THAI

Creamy Dessert Teas and Sweet Drinks
for Festive Celebration

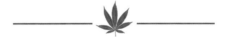

Making Hemp Milks and Coconut Milks

My chai and bhang recipes use either raw, shelled hemp seed or young or mature coconut flesh to make delicious, creamy beverages that are generally recognized as safe for many people with food allergies and sensitivities when they are produced in a clean area with no cross-contact with major allergens like dairy or tree nuts. Making hemp or coconut milk at home is the best way to enjoy the fresh flavor and the assurance of a clean preparation.

I have included my favorite milk recipes here to use with the creamy bhang and chai recipes in this chapter, but you may use any kind of "milk" you prefer with these recipes, either homemade or a commercial product. In some of these recipes, coconut milk will produce the best flavor, so I've let you know when appropriate. You may also try one of my favorite milk blends by combining half coconut and half hemp milk, too!

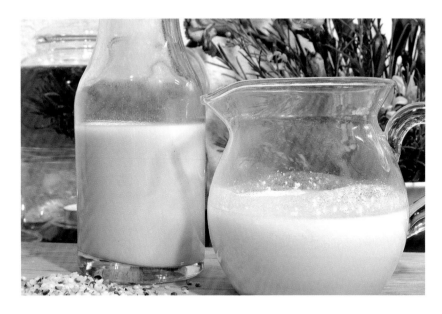

The Basic Hemp Milk Recipe

One of the most important things to remember about hemp milk and hemp seed in general, apart from it having such a wonderful flavor, is how heat-sensitive it is. Hemp milk can take a little bit of heat—but certainly not as much as coconut milk—and it does have a tendency to curdle. Hemp milk should not be heated much more than 160°F (71°C) for best results in your recipes. I like to strain my hemp milk through cheesecloth before use to remove the fiber from the seeds that have been processed into milk. Make 1 pint (480 milliliters) of hemp milk at a time and drink within 24 hours for the freshest flavor. Fresh hemp milk you make in your blender with shelled hemp seeds will last at most 2 days before it starts to sour.

1 pint (480 milliliters) cold water

¾ cup (100 grams) shelled hemp seed, or more if you prefer creamier milks

Preparation:

Blend thoroughly until milky in a blender. Strain through a cheesecloth and refrigerate or use immediately.

The Basic Coconut Milk Recipe

I like to use young coconut flesh and a little bit of coconut water to make fresh coconut milk. Young coconuts aren't available everywhere, so fresh, mature coconuts may be used along with their water inside in a blender to create coconut milk. The final concentration and creaminess of the drink is based on your preference for young or mature coconuts. Like hemp milk, you will want to strain the fiber out of the milk through cheesecloth before using or refrigerating.

When making coconut milk, work with coconut and water that is at least room temperature because coconut fats turn solid in cooler temperatures. Coconut milk is stable for at least a week when refrigerated.

1 pint (480 milliliters) warm water or warm coconut water
1 cup (175 grams) coconut (young or mature), or more if you prefer
   creamier milks

Preparation:

Blend thoroughly until milky in a blender. Strain through a cheesecloth and refrigerate or use immediately.

Cannabis Milk Infusion for Bhang and Dessert Beverages

In this chapter, cannabis is typically infused into the milk (hemp or coconut) part of our beverages before it is added to the rest of the recipe. You may use this recipe to infuse any milk of your choice, as well.

Hemp Milk Cannabis Infusion

Prepare this infusion of cannabis at lower temperatures. Unlike coconut milk, you cannot decarb cannabis directly in the milk because of the low temperature requirements (130–160°F/54°C–71°C maximum) for working with hemp milk. The best way to infuse hemp milk with the number of servings of cannabinoids that you desire is to use either the Cannabis Infusion Oil (page 11) or Tabletop Cannabis Infusion (page 33) methods described in the introductory chapter of this book, and add that to warm hemp milk before preparing chai or bhang.

Coconut Milk Cannabis Infusion

Technically, coconut milk can take much higher heat, meaning you can decarb cannabis plant material or concentrated resins and oils if you want. Your coconut milk will have a fresher taste in the final recipe if you work with the coconut milk at lower temperatures and use same method for infusing hemp milk with cannabinoids. However, you can bring this to a higher temperature than hemp milk, if you desire (above 175°F/79°C, but no more than 200°F/93°C for the best texture and flavor) when creating and serving beverages.

Masala Spice Blend

5 black peppercorns, broken
1 stick cinnamon, broken
1 green cardamom pod, broken
1 brown cardamom pod, broken
1 small thumb of fresh ginger, chopped
5 cloves
1 small piece nutmeg, broken
Pinch of fennel seed

---

2 servings of the cannabis infusion of your choice (Cannabis Infusion Oil page 11, or the Tabletop Cannabis Infusion page 33)
8 ounces (240 milliliters) water
3 teaspoons (3–4 grams) Assam, Arabic yellow label Lipton tea (Don't use any Lipton tea unless it is this one!), Red Rose brand tea (My favorite!), Irish breakfast, or another very stiff black tea—a dark, cinnamon oolong is also a nice choice for this recipe, too.
Masala spice blend (see above)
Rosewater, to splash
8 ounces (240 milliliters) hemp or coconut milk, or any milk you prefer
Jaggery sugar or other natural cane sugar cube, to sweeten

Canna-Chai Recipes

Masala Canna-Chai

Masala is the Hindi word for "spice" and means a lot of different things depending on who you ask! Masala is a mixture of spices unique to families, chefs, and regions. Here's the thing I have learned about masala: everyone's formula for masala is the right formula. Making masala for cannabis tea is as unique as you are. What flavors and experience do you seek? Here's my interpretation of the best spicy tea masala I have tried throughout the years. Makes 2 servings or a little more.

Preparation:

1. Prepare the servings of your cannabis infusion method (Cannabis Infusion Oil, page 11, or the Tabletop Cannabis Infusion, page 33) and set aside. Put the loose tea into the filter basket of your teapot and set aside.

2. Put all the spices for the blend into a pan on the stove, turn on the heat to about medium, and heat these briefly in the dry pan while stirring to release and intensify flavors—do not burn. Pour the water over them and bring to a boil. Remove from the stove and pour the water and all the spices over the tea in the filter basket. Allow this to steep for at least 2 to 5 minutes, depending on the strength of tea desired.

3. Warm the milk and add the cannabis infusion you have selected while the tea and masala are steeping. Add a splash of rosewater to the milk after you have warmed it to the desired temperature. Whisk the milk vigorously and pour into individual cups.

4. Pour the masala tea into the cups containing the milk and serve with jaggery or cane sugar cubes.

Vienna Canna–Chai

Whole Tahitian vanilla beans and gourmet Ceylon cinnamon sticks are featured in this European-inspired chai. It's a delightful and impressive after-dinner dessert beverage. Serve this to your guests at your next dinner party or event for a memorable gourmet experience.

Makes 4 servings or a little more. Ratio of tea-to-milk should be roughly half and half.

Preparation:

1. Prepare the servings of your cannabis infusion method (Cannabis Infusion Oil, page 11, or the Tabletop Cannabis Infusion, page 33) and set aside.
2. Gently warm the milk with the scraped vanilla bean paste, the whole vanilla bean, and the sugar or sweetener for 15 minutes. Remove the whole vanilla bean and whisk in the cannabis infusion you have selected.
3. Put the loose tea into the filter basket of your teapot, add the hot water, and let this steep until it is very strong, but not bitter—3 minutes or a little more. Add the warm milk to the hot tea and whisk vigorously. Pour into individual cups with one cinnamon stick in each cup. Gently stir the chai with the cinnamon stick after pouring and serve immediately.

4 servings of the cannabis infusion of your choice (Cannabis Infusion Oil page 11, or the Tabletop Cannabis Infusion page 33)

12–16 ounces (360–480 milliliters) water

5 teaspoons (5–7 grams) any high-quality black tea

12–16 ounces (360–480 milliliters) hemp or coconut milk, or any milk you prefer

1 whole vanilla bean, sliced open and scraped

4 whole Ceylon cinnamon sticks

4 teaspoons (about 17 grams) sugar, or equivalent sweetener

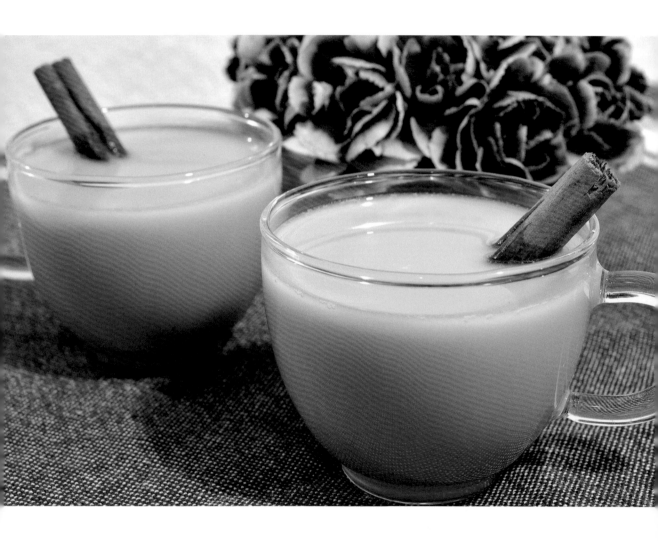

Green Dragon Lemongrass Canna-Chai

This is a really intense lemongrass and tea infusion that I make using the lemongrass I grow in my own garden. You can grow lemongrass indoors, too, if you have a sunny area. Fresh lemongrass stalks from the grocer will sprout roots almost immediately when put in soil and will continue to produce fresh stalks of lemongrass whenever you need them. Fresh lemongrass is absolutely essential to the flavor in this South Asian–inspired cannabis-infused chai. Prepare this with coconut milk for the best flavor. Makes 2 servings or a little more.

2 servings of the cannabis infusion of your choice (Cannabis Infusion Oil page 11, or the Tabletop Cannabis Infusion page 33)
8 ounces (240 milliliters) water
2 teaspoons (3 grams) matcha green tea
4 young stalks or 1 large older stalk of lemongrass, thoroughly chopped
8 ounces (240 milliliters) coconut milk, or any milk you prefer
Natural cane sugar cube or honey, to sweeten

Preparation:

1. Prepare the servings of your cannabis infusion method (Cannabis Infusion Oil, page 11, or the Tabletop Cannabis Infusion, page 33) and set aside. Whisk the matcha into a little hot water to dissolve it completely in your teapot and set aside.

2. Put the chopped lemongrass into a pan or kettle on the stove and add the water. Bring to a boil, and then pour the water and lemongrass over the tea in the filter basket of the teapot with the dissolved matcha and allow this to steep for at least 3 minutes in the matcha tea. Remove the filter basket with the lemongrass.

3. Warm the coconut milk and add the cannabis infusion you have selected. Whisk vigorously. Pour into individual cups. Whisk the matcha and lemongrass tea and add the matcha to the cups with the infused milk. Serve with cane sugar cubes or honey to sweeten.

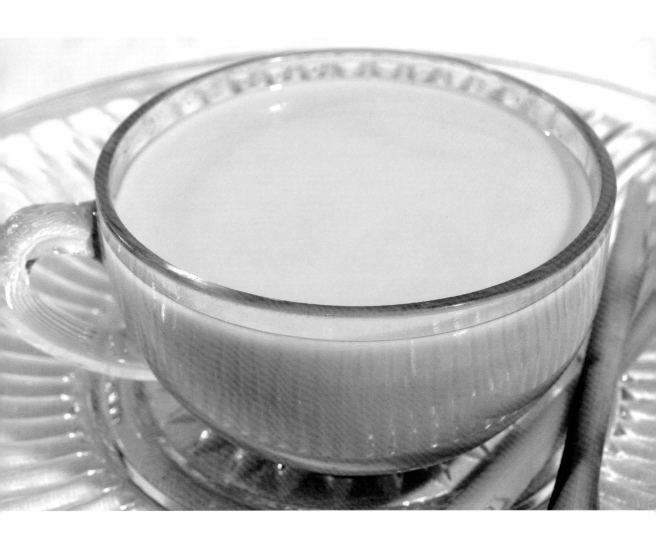

Prunus illicifolia, The Wild California Cherry You've Never Heard Of

California, land of the wild child and home of the flower children, has a native wild cherry tree that you've probably never heard of—Holly Leaf Cherry, or *Prunus illicifolia*, bears a fruit that you will never find in the supermarket. This beautiful plant teacher introduced itself to me on one of my many wildcrafting adventures. It's unique in its ability to produce a deeply floral, rose-fragranced syrup with notes of amaretto and cherry. I've never experienced anything quite like it.

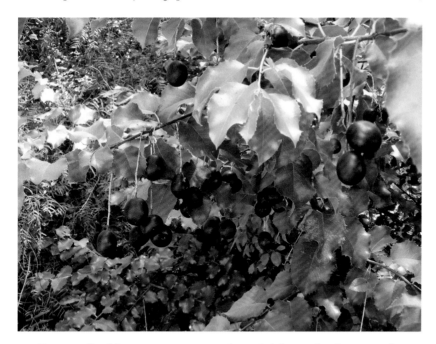

Prunus illicifolia is sometimes used in California landscaping for its drought-resistant qualities. Most people leave these cherries for the birds because they have a much larger seed, thicker skin, and thinner flesh than any commercial cherry. They are not a snacking cherry or even a pie cherry; right off of the tree, the flesh is sugar-sweet, and the skin is very chewy and slightly bitter.

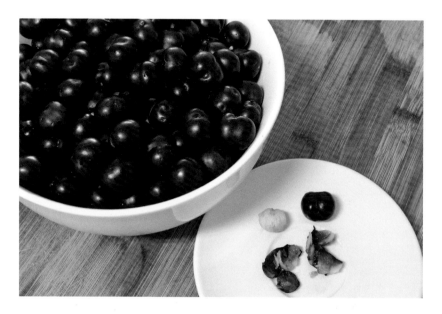

Imagine my surprise when I found these cherries on a wild trail, grabbed a few off the tree, took a few bites, and then turned around to realize the leaves of the tree were holly-shaped. I didn't really know what this tree was. I don't suggest that you do the same thing! But the good news is that the flesh and skin of this cherry, like all cherries, is safe for consumption.

The tree itself looks a little dangerous, hence the name, Holly Leaf Cherry. The easiest way to identify this tree in the wild is by the holly leaf shape of the leaves, the distinctive amaretto fragrance of the leaves when they are crushed, and the dark red to black sweet fruit that looks like a cherry or small plum. In drier and more disturbed areas, the trees will be small, almost shrub-like, with fruits that can be harvested from the ground.

I think this wild California cherry embodies so much of what California is—it's the wild child of cherries that deserves a place in your tea cup to celebrate the legalization of cannabis! This cherry is ready for harvesting in the months of August and September, just in time for the holiday season, too.

To make my delicious California Cherry Blossom Creme Canna-Chai you are going make syrup from the very ripe fruit of the *Prunus illicifolia*. Select fruit that is not wrinkled but is at the peak of ripeness when it is dark red or almost black and easily detaches from the tree. Because the flesh is so thin, 5 pounds of fruit is going to yield about a ½ to 1 cup of syrup (about 120–240 milliliters) at the end of the cooking process. No sugar or other sweetener is added to this syrup.

Wild California Cherry Syrup

Like all cherries and other stone fruits, the pits of these cherries are toxic and should not be boiled down with the flesh to make this syrup. Separating the flesh and skin from the seed is a more involved process than working with commercial cherries, which easily release their flesh from the pit.

5 pounds or more of *Prunus illicifolia* cherries (You can use less, but you will have less syrup after the final boil.)

Large pan filled with enough water to cover the cherries

Masher or other instrument to help separate the flesh and skin from the cherries

Strainer lined in cheesecloth

More water, as needed

Preparation:

1. Put all the clean cherries into a pan with enough water to cover them, and bring them to a boil.
2. Remove the cherries from the stove and allow them to soak in the hot water. The skins will crack and the flesh will separate from some of the cherries. After they have cooled, sufficiently use your masher or other instrument to rub the flesh and skin off all the pits. Remove the pits from the mash.
3. Place the mash back on the stove and bring this to a rolling boil, and then turn off the heat and allow the mash to soak for at least 1 hour.

Bring this to a rolling boil once again, and then turn off the heat and let this mash sit, covered, for at least 3 hours.

4. Using a masher, work the flesh and skins into a pulp; your liquid should be dark or wine-colored and not yet thickened. Add more water, if necessary, to complete the last boil with the flesh and skin. You will boil this down to its halfway point from where the water level started in your pan in step 3. When it reaches this point, remove the mash from the stove and allow this to cool.

5. Run the mash through the strainer lined with cheesecloth. Squeeze as much juice as you can from the cherry mash.

6. Place the dark cherry liquid back on the stove and begin a gentle simmering process until it reaches the syrup stage. Watch this carefully and stir frequently so that it does not burn! This is called the thread stage; the liquid will concentrate the cherry sugars so that it has a similar consistency to maple syrup. Typically, the temperature range of your cherry syrup will be about 215°F (101°C) at this stage. Remove this from the stove and let it cool briefly before pouring into a sealed glass jar. Allow this to cool to room temperature before refrigerating.

7. Refrigeration is a must! The syrup develops its unique rose floral profile after refrigeration for a few days and continues to "blossom" with even stronger floral fragrance over time. The syrup is ready to use after a few days to one week of refrigeration when you can open the jar and immediately detect this fine floral fragrance. This syrup should be kept in refrigeration and used within 45 days.

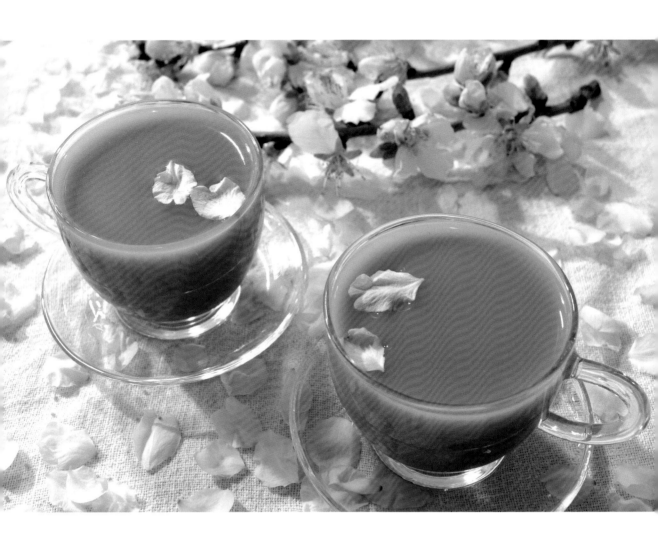

California Cherry Blossom Creme Canna-Chai

2 servings of the cannabis infusion of your choice (Cannabis Infusion Oil page 11, or the Tabletop Cannabis Infusion page 33)

8 ounces (240 milliliters) boiling water

2 teaspoons (3–4 grams) black or golden tea

8 ounces (240 milliliters) hemp or coconut milk, or any milk you prefer

1–3 teaspoons (5–15 milliliters) or more Wild California Cherry Syrup (page 116) OR your favorite cherry syrup with a splash of rosewater

This is my favorite canna-chai recipe! The magnificent syrup of the Holly Leaf Cherry makes this chai creamy, floral, and fruity. It is an impressive beverage to celebrate legalization, the holidays, or just to treat yourself to something really special for getting out there in the wild and harvesting this very special cherry. Makes 2 servings or a little more.

Regarding the tea to use for this recipe, my preferences are either 2 large or 4 small black pearls or golden monkey tea. For a really unique flavor experience, prepare this with milk oolong and skip the milk infusion here by adding the cannabis infusion of your choice directly to the tea.

Preparation:

1. Prepare the servings of your cannabis infusion method (Cannabis Infusion Oil, page 11, or the Tabletop Cannabis Infusion, page 33) and set aside. Put the loose tea into the filter basket of your teapot and set aside.

2. Bring the water to a boil on the stove and pour over the tea in the filter basket. Allow this to steep for at least 3 minutes.

3. Warm the milk and add the cannabis infusion you have selected. You may add the cherry syrup directly to the milk now. Whisk vigorously and pour into individual cups.

4. When the tea has finished steeping, pour it into the cups with the sweet milk, whisk, and serve with cherry blossom garnishes as an extra touch for a special occasion.

Here's a tip for making a fabulous Cherry Blossom Crème Canna-Chai If you don't have access to these unique California cherries: Substitute your favorite cherry syrup or preserves and add a splash of rosewater!

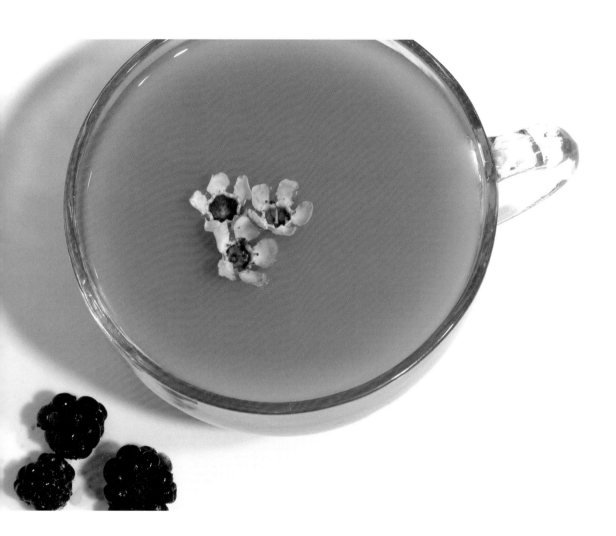

More Creamy Canna-Chai and Bhang Recipes From My Kitchen

Assam and Blackberry Blossom Canna-Chai

2 servings of the cannabis infusion of your choice (Cannabis Infusion Oil page 11, or the Tabletop Cannabis Infusion page 33)

10 ounces (300 milliliters) water

6 ounces (180 milliliters) coconut milk

2 teaspoons (3 grams) Assam or another rich, black tea like Irish breakfast

5 or more dried blackberry blossoms

10 fresh, frozen, or sun-dried blackberries

Sweetener of your choice

Assam is a rich and dark tea that makes a perfect cup of milky chai. When this favorite tea of India and Pakistan is paired with fruit and florals with deep flavors like the wild Himalayan blackberry blossoms and fruit, the results are always divine.

In the late summer, I pick the berries, both ripe and shriveled. I like to freeze the ripe berries and sun dry and store the shriveled ones. Wild berries and other wild fruits in California tend to concentrate their flavors densely due to the lack of rainfall in the summer months. These highly concentrated flavors are desirable when making a fruity/floral chai like this one; grocery store blackberries are not at all like these. Makes 2 servings, or a little more.

Preparation:

1. Prepare the servings of your cannabis infusion method (Cannabis Infusion Oil, page 11, or the Tabletop Cannabis Infusion, page 33) and set aside. Put the loose tea and blackberry blossoms into the filter basket of your teapot and set aside.

2. Put the blackberries in a pan on the stove with the water and bring to a boil. Squeeze and break them before pouring the water and berries over the tea and blossoms for steeping. Steep for at least 3 minutes.

3. Warm the coconut milk and add the cannabis infusion. Whisk vigorously and pour into individual cups. Add the tea when it is finished steeping. This chai is best when it's generously sweetened, but your tastes may vary. Sweeten to your liking and serve.

Thai Iced Canna-Tea

Thai iced tea is a favorite sweet tea beverage for the unique spice blend as well as the deep red-orange color that looks so pretty in the glass when milk is added. The Thai spice blend I use is totally artisanal—no packaged Thai tea with artificial colorings. The beautiful color of this tea comes from three sources: Ceylon tea, which is known for its deep red color; sassafras bark; and turmeric root. All three of these ingredients lend their unique flavors to this tea to create the Thai tea flavor you're familiar with. You'll be making a very concentrated base of tea, which will need to be refrigerated first before serving. Makes 2 servings.

Spice Blend
½ vanilla bean, chopped
1 large star anise
½ teaspoon (1 gram) sassafras bark
1 small turmeric root, chopped
1 small thumb ginger, chopped

_____

2 servings of the cannabis infusion of your choice (Cannabis Infusion Oil page 11, or the Tabletop Cannabis Infusion page 33)
8 ounces (240milliliters) water
10 ounces (300 milliliters) coconut milk
4 teaspoons (4–5 grams) Ceylon red tea
4 or more teaspoons (15 grams) sugar or xylitol, or more if you would like this tea to be super-sweet
Ice

Preparation:

1. Prepare the servings of your cannabis infusion method (Cannabis Infusion Oil, page 11, or the Tabletop Cannabis Infusion, page 33). Warm the coconut milk just enough to thoroughly dissolve the sugar and the cannabis infusion while whisking. Set aside and allow to cool to room temperature while you prepare the tea.

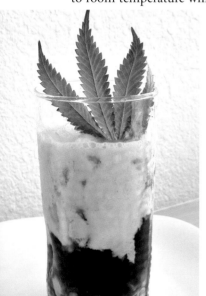

2. In a pan on the stove, add the spices to the water. Bring this to a boil, take it off of the heat, add the tea, and let it steep for at least 5 minutes or more before straining, cooling to room temperature, and then refrigerating. Allow this to cool for at least 20 minutes or longer in the refrigerator.

3. Set up your glasses and fill with ice. Pour the tea over the ice in equal amounts into each glass. Now whisk and pour the sweetened cannabis coconut milk over the ice and serve immediately with a straw.

Coconut Matcha Bhang

2 servings of the cannabis infusion of your choice (Cannabis Infusion Oil page 11, or the Tabletop Cannabis Infusion page 33)

12 ounces (360 milliliters) fresh coconut milk

2 teaspoons (3 grams) of any grade matcha

2 tablespoons (30 milliliters) hot water

Coconut sugar or cane sugar, to sweeten

Matcha can be quite expensive, and when it comes to using matcha for culinary purposes, an everyday culinary grade will do for this recipe. I've used both culinary and ceremonial grade to make this bhang, and I have to say that a really high grade of matcha is not necessary for delicious flavor—an everyday grade will certainly do. This is a tasty and oh-so-easy bhang that can be made to impress without a lot of fuss. Makes 2 servings.

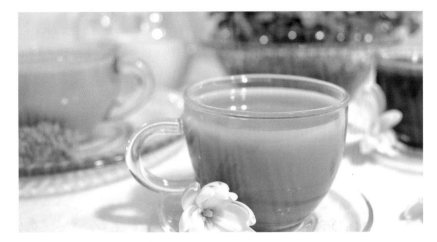

Preparation:

1. Prepare the servings of your cannabis infusion method (Cannabis Infusion Oil, page 11, or the Tabletop Cannabis Infusion, page 33) and set aside. Thoroughly dissolve the matcha in the hot water.

2. Put the fresh coconut milk in a blender with the matcha and blend for about 30 seconds. Transfer this to a pan on the stove and warm gently. Vigorously whisk in the sugar and the cannabis infusion of your choice.

3. Remove from the stove and whisk the warm bhang again before pouring into individual cups and serving.

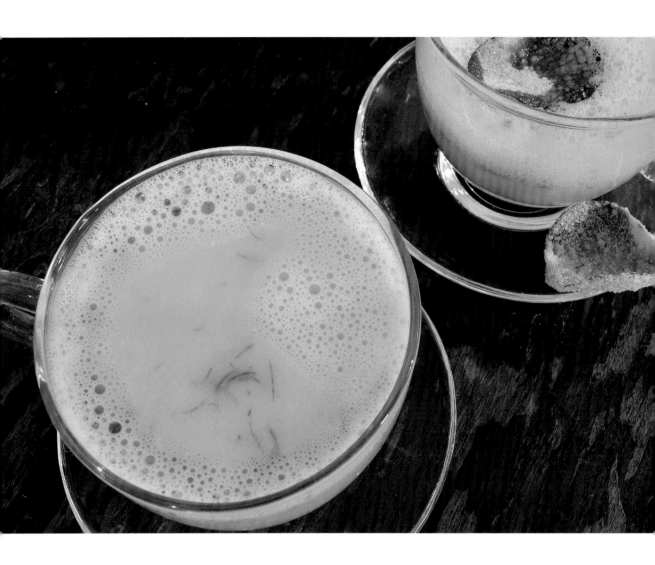

Saffron Rose Bhang

2 servings of the cannabis
    infusion of your choice
    (Cannabis Infusion
    Oil page 11, or the
    Tabletop Cannabis
    Infusion page 33)
12 ounces (360 milliliters)
    coconut or hemp milk,
    or any milk you prefer
20 or more threads saffron
1 tablespoon (15
    milliliters) rosewater
2 teaspoons (10 grams)
    sugar or xylitol

I fell in love with Saffron as a singular tisane flavor after learning about this from my local Afghani grocer, who taught me how to buy the best saffron (Afghan-sourced was his favorite, of course!). This saffron and rose bhang is the perfect beverage for curling up on a rainy afternoon with a book of Rumi's poetry. Garnish with rose petal terpene entourage from chapter 1. Makes 2 servings.

Preparation:

1. Prepare the servings of your cannabis infusion method (Cannabis Infusion Oil, page 11, or the Tabletop Cannabis Infusion, page 33) and set aside.

2. Slowly warm the milk you select with the threads of saffron and your cannabis infusion selection. You're going to want to hold the milk at around 160°F (71°C) for at least 10 minutes to fully infuse the saffron into the milk. For the most intense flavor, I add the saffron to the cold milk and let that sit on the counter infusing for 15 minutes before heating it, adding the cannabis infusion, and then maintaining the low heat above for at least 10 minutes to further infuse the saffron flavor and color.

3. Add the sugar and whisk in before removing from the heat. Add the tablespoon of rosewater and whisk vigorously before pouring into cups and serving.

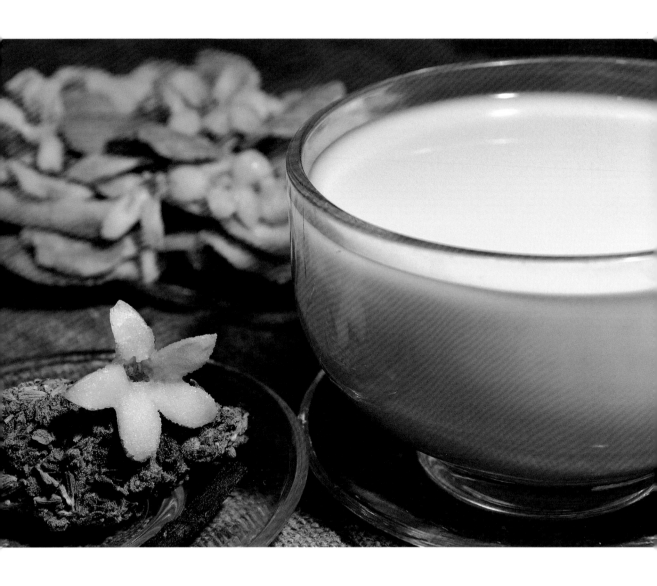

Sweet Island Bhang

2 servings of the cannabis infusion of your choice (Cannabis Infusion Oil page 11, or the Tabletop Cannabis Infusion page 33)

12 ounces (360 milliliters) coconut milk

½ vanilla bean, chopped

1 thumb ginger, chopped

1 small turmeric root, chopped

1 tablespoon (15 milliliters) orange flower water

3 teaspoons (15 grams) sugar or xylitol

Powdered nutmeg, to garnish

This is for coconut and tropical flavor lovers everywhere. If you can get access to fresh jasmine or citrus blossoms, I would highly recommend them as a fragrant garnish to complete the flavor of this creamy bhang. Makes 2 servings.

Preparation:

1. Prepare the servings of your cannabis infusion method (Cannabis Infusion Oil, page 11, or the Tabletop Cannabis Infusion, page 33) and set aside.

2. Slowly warm the milk on the stove and hold the milk at around 160°F (71°C) for at least 10 minutes to fully infuse the spices into the milk. Strain out the whole spices and whisk in your cannabis infusion selection.

3. Whisk in the sugar before removing the bhang from the heat. Add the orange flower water and whisk vigorously. Serve in cups and garnish with a little nutmeg powder and jasmine or citrus blossoms.

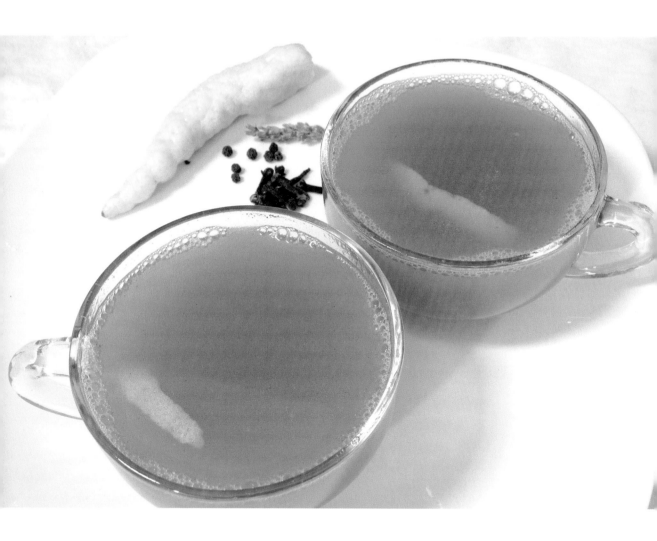

Entertain With These Delightful Cannabis-Infused Beverages

Laughing Buddha Mulled Canna–Cider

Fruit and Spice Mulling Blend

¼ cup (40 grams) Buddha's hand citron, chopped
5 black peppercorns
2 cinnamon sticks
3 green cardamom pods, cracked open
8 clove buds
3 whole allspice
1 teaspoon (0.50 grams) lavender flowers
1 large thumb ginger, chopped
Dash of nutmeg or nutmeg pieces

_____

4 servings of the cannabis infusion of your choice (Cannabis Infusion Oil page 11, or the Tabletop Cannabis Infusion page 33)
Fruit and spice mulling blend (see above)
24 ounces (720 milliliters) fresh-pressed apple cider
Cut Buddha's hand citron, for garnish

If you need a cannabis beverage to impress during the holiday season, this mulled canna-cider is jolly and will bring much joy and luck to your holiday celebration! The special ingredient in this mulled cider, the Buddha's hand citron, is a specialty citrus typically available only during the holiday season—so if you plan on making this cider any time, cut the citron and store it in tightly closed bags or containers in your freezer so the flavor is preserved. This recipe makes 4 (6-ounce or 180-milliliter) servings, but you can adjust the ingredients based on the number of people you are serving.

Preparation:

1. Prepare the servings of your cannabis infusion method (Cannabis Infusion Oil, page 11, or the Tabletop Cannabis Infusion, page 33) and set aside.
2. Heat the cider until steam rises, and then pour over the spices in the mulling pot or teapot. Gently warm your cider with the spices over a low heat or in a teapot with a tea candle for 20 minutes or more, covered.
3. Remove the filter holding the spices or strain them from the cider. Vigorously whisk in the cannabis infusion. This can be served immediately or left to warm, and whisked again before serving. Garnish before serving! Spices may be used to infuse 2 or more pots of cider before discarding.

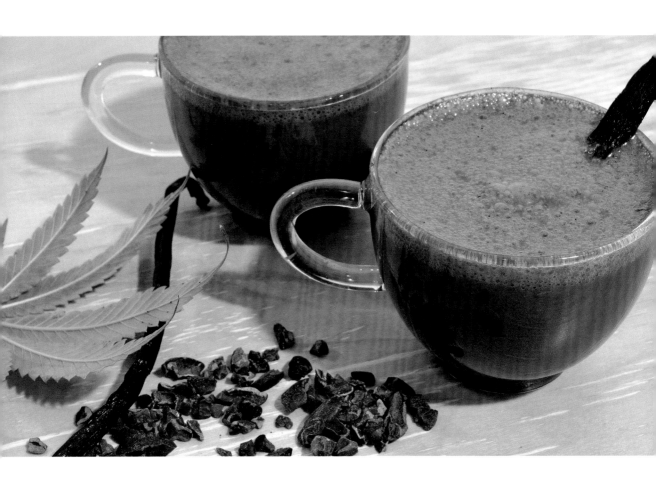

Shaman's Tasting Chocolates

Cannabis can be a shamanic experience. If you think you're ready for that, this tasting chocolate is designed to be served with cannabis infusions rich in cannabinoids. I'm not just talking about THC, but CBD, too, can be a shamanic experience of deep healing and contemplation.

I have two recipes for this tasting chocolate: one is a black forest–inspired cherry vanilla tasting chocolate that is incredible with CBD infusions, and the other is a very spicy pepper and ginger tasting chocolate for infusions with soaring THC percentages that can best be described as "blasting off!" Please use the guide in the introductory chapter when calculating the THC or CBD levels that are best for you and your guests.

The Black Forest CBD Healer Chocolate

Makes 2 servings or more.

2 or more servings of the cannabis CBD infusion of your choice (Cannabis Infusion Oil page 11, or the Tabletop Cannabis Infusion page 33)

16 ounces (480 milliliters) coconut or hemp milk, or any milk you prefer

1½ tablespoons (9 grams) powdered cacao

1 whole vanilla bean, scraped

15 dried, canned, or fresh sour cherries

1–2 tablespoons (15–30 grams) sugar or xylitol, or more, depending on the level of sweetness you prefer

Preparation:

1. Prepare the servings of your cannabis infusion method (Cannabis Infusion Oil, page 11, or the Tabletop Cannabis Infusion, page 33) and set aside.
2. In a blender, add the milk, cherries, chocolate, vanilla paste, and sugar, and blend until smooth. Transfer to a pan on the stove and gently heat to 160°F (71°C) while whisking in the cannabis infusion.
3. Remove from the heat, whisk vigorously, and serve immediately. Garnish with whipped cream, if desired and on hand.

The Shaman's Launch Pad Chocolate

Makes 2 or more servings.

Preparation:

1. Prepare the servings of your cannabis infusion method (Cannabis Infusion Oil, page 11, or the Tabletop Cannabis Infusion, page 33) and set aside.
2. In a pan on the stove, warm the milk with the hot peppers, ginger, vanilla, chocolate, and sugar for 10 minutes at 160°F (71°C), until thoroughly infused.
3. Strain the plant material from the milk and whisk in the cannabis infusion vigorously over the heat. Remove from the heat and serve immediately. Garnish with a small cannabis leaf, if desired.

2 servings of the cannabis infusion of your choice (Cannabis Infusion Oil page 11, or the Tabletop Cannabis Infusion page 33)

16 ounces (480 milliliters) coconut or hemp milk, or any milk you prefer

2 tablespoons (12 grams) powdered cacao

½ vanilla bean, scraped

1 thumb of fresh ginger, grated, or 1 teaspoon ginger powder

4 or 5 whole, dried Chinese red pepper pods, or cayenne pepper pods

1–2 tablespoons (15–30) grams sugar or xylitol, or more, depending on the level of sweetness you prefer

Emerald Triangle/Pineapple Express Wedding Punch

Who spiked the wedding punch?! That fizzy, fruity, sweet, and very innocent-looking wedding punch with floating sherbet is the traditional American-style cold punch served at weddings and showers—sometimes spiked with a little rum, depending on the social function.

My punch is definitely spiked, but not with rum! This punch uses the Tabletop Cannabis Infusion method from the introductory chapter (page 33) for the best results and is also dairy-free.

Instead of sherbet, this punch is paired with dairy-free coconut ice cream to float on top. Remember to label the punchbowl at your gathering so no one is surprised! Double or triple this recipe based on the number of guests who will want to enjoy a wedding punch infused with the finest cannabis from the Emerald Triangle.

Note that you can make another version of this recipe aptly named the Pineapple Express that pairs beautifully with dairy-free strawberry coconut ice cream. Keep in mind that matcha tea is the secret ingredient that will give this pineapple punch a lovely emerald color and bright floral flavors.

For Emerald Triangle

5 or more servings of the Tabletop Cannabis Infusion (page 33)

2 quarts (2 liters) good-quality ginger ale

2 cups (480 milliliters) pear juice

1 cup (240 milliliters) sour cherry or blackberry juice

1 pint of vanilla or mango coconut ice cream (dairy-free) to float on punch

For Pineapple Express

5 or more servings of the Tabletop Cannabis Infusion (page 33)

2 quarts (2 liters) good-quality ginger ale

3 cups (720 milliliters) pineapple juice

1 tablespoon (6–8 grams) matcha green tea

1 pint of strawberry coconut ice cream (dairy-free) to float on punch

Preparation:

1. All the ingredients should be ice cold before starting! Gently warm 1 cup (240 milliliters) of the juice on the stove and vigorously whisk in the Tabletop Cannabis Infusion (page 33) that you have already prepared and set aside for this recipe. If you are making the Pineapple Express punch, whisk in the matcha green tea along with the cannabis infusion. Thoroughly whisk the warm juice into the rest of the cold juice. A blender is very effective for bringing the warm cannabis-infused juice together with the cold juice quickly. If there is any delay in making the punch, the juice should be whisked, shaken, or blended again before adding to the punchbowl for best results.

2. In a punch bowl, add all the juice and slowly pour in the cold ginger ale while whisking.

3. Float small scoops of the coconut or mango/coconut ice cream for the Emerald triangle version or strawberry coconut ice cream for the Pineapple Express version, and serve.

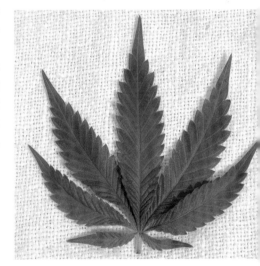

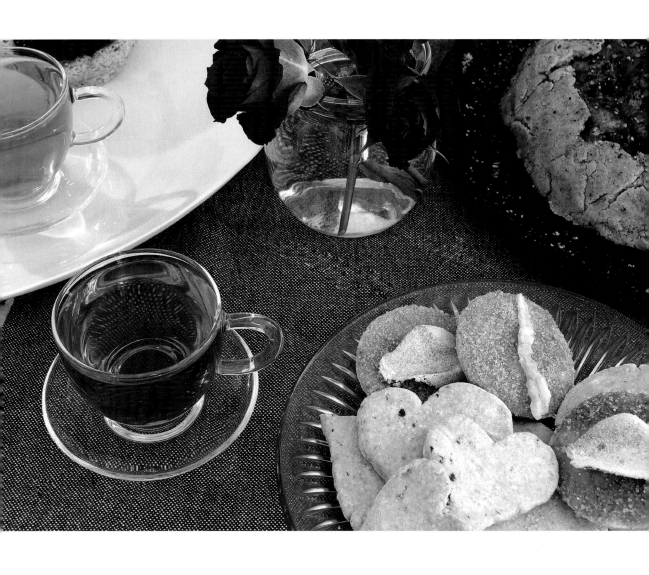

CHAPTER FIVE

CANNABIS-INFUSED BEVERAGE AND SENSITIVITY CUISINE PAIRINGS FOR BRUNCH, LUNCH, OR ANYTIME

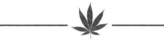

A Word on Sensitivity Cuisine and Pairing with Cannabis-Infused Beverage

When I began putting the recipes from my sensitivity kitchen into this book, I selected the ones most loved in my kitchen to pair with cannabis beverage and broth. I would be honored above all for you to find as much bliss in the flavors and culinary style in this book as the guests in my own kitchen have!

Sensitivity cuisine is a term I coined to describe a simple culinary practice: cuisine that is free of all the big eight allergens (wheat (including gluten), soy, tree nuts, peanuts, eggs, shellfish, fish, dairy), or the big nine allergens (all of the big eight plus sesame), or the big fourteen international allergens (all of the big eight plus celery, sesame, lupin, mollusks, sulphites, mustard), plus any additional ingredients selected by the chef. So what are the big eight, big nine, and big fourteen exactly? These are the foods that have been identified as the causes of most of all allergic reactions globally.[5]

My personal journey with life-threatening anaphylaxis and food allergies has been one of both pain and discovery. My first anaphylactic events started as a toddler. I have both allergies and autoimmune disease, which are both birth defects in my immune system. I am grateful for the doctors and my EpiPens, but I am also grateful for the wonderful healing and soothing properties of cannabis that have made my journey with immune system disorder much more comfortable in the years that I have had my medical marijuana card.

My array of food allergies includes eggs, yeast, insect, and many agricultural funguses. That excludes a lot of foods—I'm often asked by stunned chefs and new friends what exactly I can eat! I don't view my food allergies as "do nots," but rather as a starting point for discovery and innovation. I am reminded of nineteenth-century chemist Alfred Bird and his wife, Elizabeth, who had the same food allergies that I have (eggs and yeast). Bird made many contributions to the world of modern baking on behalf of his wife. He invented a yeast-free baking powder in 1843 for her—the same baking powder used by chefs and bakers all over the world today would not exist if it were not for the food allergies of Mrs. Bird![6] Alfred Bird's culinary discoveries are a cornerstone of modern, quick pastry and baking.

---

5   *Food Allergies: What You Need to Know*
    http://www.fda.gov/Food/ResourcesForYou/Consumers/ucm079311.htm
    Food Allergy Facts
    http://allergytraining.food.gov.uk/english/food-allergy-facts.aspx
6   What's Cooking America—*History of Baking Powder*:
    https://whatscookingamerica.net/History/BakingPowderHistory.htm.
    Royal Pharmaceutical Society of Great Britain—*Pharmacy the Mother of Invention*:
    http://www.rpsgb.org/informationresources/museum/exhibitions/themotherofinvention/

In my sensitivity kitchen, I exclude the big nine allergens plus fungus and fermentation, which includes aged foods and beverage. All the recipes in this book follow this method of sensitivity cuisine. Ingredients are always fresh and very clean. You'll want to wash your fresh fruits and vegetables well and discard any fruit or vegetable with mold or age. I'm a fan of the soapberry. These are perfect for tossing into a bucket of room-temperature water and suds-ing up to wash fruits and vegetables. Flours should be tightly sealed and kept in the freezer with a moisture-absorbing pack. Fresh food should be prepared and eaten quickly—within a day or two. Rice and grains are carefully examined for insects and debris. Washed grains are preferred. Farmers' markets are almost always better than supermarkets when it comes to fresh food.

Sorghum, GABA sweet brown rice, and teff are the whole grains used in these pastry recipes for their wheat-like qualities for building a rich pastry or quick bread. Arrowroot is a starchy root powder made from a tropical plant and is the finishing ingredient also essential to the texture, binding, and structure. Only authentic arrowroot, *Maranta arundinacea*, is recommended for best results. And last, but not least, my pastry creations also use aquafaba, otherwise known as bean juice. This juice provides an egg-like structure and is the liquid that can be obtained from a can of chickpeas or white beans or from cooking these beans from scratch. I find that organic canned beans in cans free of BPA linings are a reliable and quick source of aquafaba. Made in this way, these gluten-free and major allergen-free pastries have good texture and structure without the need for gums like xanthan.

Arrowroot: A Staple Ingredient of Sensitivity Cuisine

Arrowroot is a favorite ingredient in my sensitivity kitchen—and one that doesn't get enough attention in most cooking circles, in my opinion. Sure, you may be familiar with this ingredient for making stir-fry, or crisping fries, or as an ingredient in teething biscuits for babies—but, did you know that arrowroot was a favorite ingredient in nineteenth-century cooking for everyone of sensitive constitution, including babies? Arrowroot is one of the most hypoallergenic and easily digested food ingredients known to mankind.

When most chefs think of arrowroot, its role as a supporting ingredient come to mind, but, in the nineteenth century recipes that called for this ingredient, arrowroot was at center stage. For example, arrowroot biscuits were *arrowroot* biscuits with wheat or rice in the supportive role. How far we have come today when most commercially available arrowroot biscuits are manufactured with mostly grain and cheaper, starchy substitutes for authentic arrowroot? Arrowroot was not just for the ailing, but a beautiful ingredient with a delightful texture and satisfying crisp. It is a delicious and easily digested food for the medical marijuana patient recovering from illness today, just as it was for medical marijuana patients of the nineteenth century—truly a staple ingredient for your artisanal sensitivity kitchen. Get rid of the little container-sized arrowroot powder in your spice rack and opt for a sack of arrowroot powder to make these recipes featuring this fabulous ingredient!

Arrowroot Tea Biscuit for Cannabis Entourage Tea or Tisane

My everyday arrowroot biscuit to enjoy with tea can be served on any occasion or time of day. You can serve these plain with cannabis tea or decorate them with sugar and terpene entourage herbs and fruits from chapter 1. You could also flavor it however you'd like, so feel free to incorporate vanilla scraped from half a whole vanilla bean, some crushed lavender or rose petals, a dash of crushed jasmine tea leaves (or any tea leaves), ginger, citron, etc.

This arrowroot biscuit is very crisp and holds up well in tea—designed for dunking as much as you like, this cookie doesn't crumble. After baking,

⅓ cup (80 milliliters) aquafaba (or more if necessary to add moisture to the dough)

⅓ cup (80 milliliters) coconut oil

Pinch of black salt for flavor (kala namak)

¼ teaspoon (1 gram) salt

Any selection of flavors you would like to add to the dough like a scraped vanilla bean (see above for more ideas)

Splash of rose or orange flower or rosewater water, if desired

½ cup (100 grams) sugar

1¼ cup (175 grams) sorghum flour

⅔ cup (88 grams) + 3 tablespoons (27 grams) arrowroot powder

¼ teaspoon (1 gram) baking powder

Extra arrowroot for rolling out the dough

Sugar and/or terpene entourage, for decoration

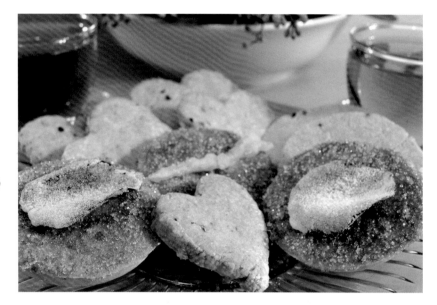

you'll want to seal up these biscuits in a closed container so that they do not become overly hard.

Try this tea biscuit rolled out about bit thicker than pie crust for the best crunch and dunk! Makes about 24 biscuits.

Preparation:

1. Combine aquafaba, coconut oil, black salt, salt, floral water, and the scraped paste from the vanilla bean (if you'd like to create a vanilla-flavored biscuit) in one bowl. In another bowl combine the dry ingredients, sugar, sorghum flour, arrowroot, baking powder, and any dry herbs you have selected like crushed rose petals, lavender, or tea leaves.

2. Add the dry ingredients to the liquid ingredients a little bit at a time until you are able to work the dough into a ball that can be rolled out. Use a little more arrowroot if necessary to stiffen the dough. Use more

aquafaba and culinary floral water if necessary to moisten the dough and bring it together.

3. Cover the dough and chill in the refrigerator for at least 10 minutes. Preheat the oven to 350°F (177°C) while the dough chills. Grease your cookie pan with a little bit of coconut oil, if needed.

4. Set up your counter with a rolling pin and board. Sprinkle some arrow-root on the surface where you'll be rolling out the dough. Form the dough into a ball, press down on the rolling surface, and then roll out to approximately ¼ of an inch (6 millimeters) or a little less. Use a cookie cutter or knife to cut the biscuits out in whatever shape you'd like. If the dough becomes dry, or you need to roll it again, sprinkle it with aquafaba to moisten. You may also sprinkle or lightly spray the biscuits with a culinary floral water before baking.

5. Bake for about 15 minutes at 350°F (177° C). Cool on a plate for 20 minutes and then seal in a container until you're ready to decorate or serve to maintain freshness for up to two weeks.

Decorate and Sweeten

These arrowroot biscuits are subtle, lightly sweet, and great with cannabis tea or tisane just as they are. But they are also a delightful canvas for even more sweetness and flavor when you decorate them with sugar and terpene entourage herbs and fruits.

Lightly paint the surface of the biscuit with a mixture of one part acacia gum, and one part any flavored liquid you prefer, such as rosewater or tea. Sprinkle decorative sugar as desired. Affix terpene entourage herbs or fruits with a drop of the thick acacia gum liquid you have prepared. Dry in a warm oven, 200°F (93°C), for about 10 minutes. Seal in a container for storage up to two weeks or serve right away.

Arrowroot Trio: Tasting Crackers, Savory Rustic Crackers, and Breadstick for Cannabis Entourage Broth

⅓ cup (80 milliliters) aquafaba (or more if necessary to add moisture to the dough)

⅓ cup (80 milliliters) rice bran oil (if you're making the Tasting Crackers), olive oil, or coconut oil

½ teaspoon (2 grams) salt

¼ teaspoon (1 gram) baking powder for the Tasting Crackers or the Breadsticks

OR

½ teaspoon (2 grams) baking powder for the Savory Rustic Crackers

⅔ cup (88 grams) arrowroot powder

1 cup (140 grams) sorghum flour

Spices or seasonings of your choice

A very similar, yet savory version of the arrowroot tea biscuit. This recipe will make three different treats, depending on what you would like to serve. The Tasting Cracker is a plain cracker perfect for clearing the palate while tasting tea, broth, or even wine. The Savory Rustic Cracker is a flavored flatbread cracker you can top with anything! And the crisp Breadstick is the perfect accompaniment for any of the savory cannabis broth and entourage recipes in chapter 3 of this book. It's a great canvas for any flavor you would like to create and makes a fine dunking breadstick that doesn't turn to mush.

To make the Tasting Cracker, use the basic recipe here, which only contains salt, and roll out about as thick as a pie crust before cutting into

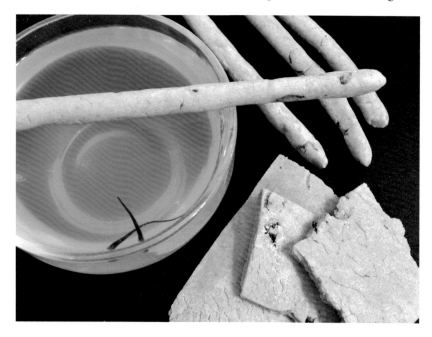

any shape you want. To make the Savory Rustic Crackers, add double the amount of baking powder to the recipe and roll it out just a bit thinner than the Tasting Crackers.

To make the breadsticks, use the standard recipe for the Tasting Crackers and add whatever seasonings you would like. Dry cured olives, rosemary, garlic, whole toasted hemp seed, and sun-dried tomatoes are among my favorite additions to the Savory Crackers or Breadsticks, which can be rolled in coarse salt and a little black pepper before baking. Remember to chop fresh herbs or spices finely before adding to the dough.

The basic dough for these recipes is made with rice bran oil, olive oil, or coconut oil, depending on which you're making. The tasting crackers are always made with rice bran oil so the flavor is very neutral; the Savory Crackers and Breadsticks can be made with the oil of your choice. Makes 12 to 24 crackers or breadsticks.

Preparation:

1. Combine aquafaba, oil (rice bran, olive, or coconut), and salt in a bowl. Combine the dry ingredients of baking powder, arrowroot, sorghum, any additional seasonings you would like, and baking powder in a separate bowl. Add the dry ingredients to the wet ingredients until you are able to work the dough into a ball that can be rolled out. You may need to sprinkle more aquafaba on the dough as you knead to keep it pliable while rolling out.

2. Cover the dough and chill in the refrigerator for at least 10 minutes. Preheat the oven to 350°F (177°C) while the dough chills. Grease your cookie sheet with a little bit of the oil you used to make the crackers or breadsticks—rice bran oil, olive oil, or coconut oil—if needed.

3. *For the crackers:* Roll out on a flat surface to about the thickness of a pie crust or thinner. *For the breadsticks:* Pinch off a thumb-sized piece of dough. As you begin to roll this in your hands, keep in mind this is gluten-free dough and may have a tendency to break while rolling—just

pinch the dough back together as you roll into sticks on a flat surface. Your breadsticks should be thin and long. Once the sticks are finished baking (next step), they will retain their breadstick shape perfectly. Roll with cracked pepper, coarse salt, or any other spice you prefer before baking.

4. Bake for about 15 to 20 minutes at 350°F (177° C). Cool on a plate for 20 minutes and then seal in a container to maintain freshness for up to two weeks or until you are ready to embellish or serve.

Embellish with Flavor

You can embellish these breadsticks with spice-coated terpene entourages for the savory cannabis broths in chapter 3 and create quite the impressive service with these broths. Use one part acacia gum and one part water as an adhesive—a few drops is all that's required. Dry in the oven for 10 minutes at 200°F (93°C).

Good Vibrations for Good Libations: The Art of the GABA Pastry

I believe cannabis beverages are optimized not only when some of their terpene entourages are reintroduced, but also when they're paired with non-medicated cuisine that emphasizes the positive effects of the cannabinoids in the beverage.

GABA pastry is the ideal complementary cuisine for cannabis tea-time, as it is both delicious and soothing. All varieties of tea are rich in GABA, as well!

What is GABA and GABA pastry? GABA, otherwise known as *gamma*-Aminobutyric acid, is an inhibitory neurotransmitter responsible for many functions in the nervous system. In the simplest layman's terms, it is primarily a relaxing, anti-anxiety neurotransmitter. GABA pastry is a pastry or quick bread created from sweet brown rice that has been germinated over twenty-four to forty-eight hours to form GABA. It is then turned into a batter or dough and combined with other grains or seeds to create the desired pastry or quick bread, such as a pie shell, biscuit, or cake.

GABA rice, otherwise known as germinated brown rice, has a rich nutritional profile that has been noted in scientific literature[7] for its superior taste and texture, as well as high content of the desirable *gamma*-Aminobutyric acid. GABA pastry is a staple in my kitchen, and it's a delicious ingredient to prepare many recipes for sensitivity cuisine. It is free of all major allergens and is easy to digest, making this a great food for medical marijuana patients. GABA is also a great pairing for recreational cannabis consumption! GABA can help soothe those moments of cannabis overindulgence.

The three basic ingredients in the GABA pastry and quick bread recipe include GABA sweet brown rice, sorghum or teff flour, and arrowroot powder. Leavening is accomplished with one or more of the following: baking powder, baking soda, vinegar, and seltzer water. Binding and increased flexibility is achieved using aquafaba. GABA sweet brown rice has all the wonderful benefits of germination, which include an increase in protein as well as superb stickiness and binding qualities that lend themselves to building a nice pastry or bread structure.

How to Make Germinated GABA Sweet Brown Rice

Making GABA sweet brown rice is a simple process that takes at least 12 hours in warmer temperatures and is best when it is allowed to germinate for 24 to 48 hours. You may have seen the elaborate new rice cookers on

1–2 cups (about 200 grams) sweet brown rice
Warm water (105°F/41°C) to cover the rice at level
Fresh seltzer water

---

7   "Germinated brown rice as a value added rice product: A review." *Journal of Food Science Technology* (November–December 2011) 48(6):661–667 https://www.ncbi.nlm.nih.gov/pmc/articles/PMC3551059/pdf/13197_2011 _Article_232.pdf

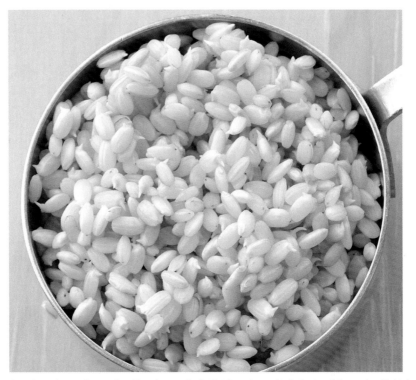

Germinated sweet brown rice. Note the small tails that have formed to indicate a living grain with high amounts of GABA.

the market that have what is called a GABA setting. This setting holds the rice grains at just over 100°F (38°C) for about 4 hours before cooking. You *do not* want to use a rice cooker like this to prepare the rice for GABA pastry. The length of time you set on these rice cookers to prepare GABA rice is not long enough to germinate the rice to the point that it has a little root tail formation—which is exactly what we want for making a good GABA pastry batter.

The process for germinating the rice does not require much in the way of special attention or tools—just time. I typically prepare my GABA sweet brown rice over the period of 24 hours with some of that time spent in a warm and sunny windowsill. As soon as you start to see the little tails appear on the grains of rice, it's ready—and bursting with GABA!

I make a few cups of the rice in advance and freeze the unused batter to use in other recipes later. This way, I always have plenty of GABA rice batter on hand to make pastries whenever I want without having to wait a day or two for the rice to germinate.

Note: *Do not substitute regular brown rice.* Sweet brown rice has the structural qualities necessary to hold together the alternative grains, starches, and seeds used in sensitivity cuisine flours like sorghum, teff, and arrowroot.

Preparation:

1. Rinse the rice in warm water several times until the water runs clear and the rice is very clean.
2. Cover the rice in warm water and allow it to stand on the counter or in a warm and sunny windowsill. Rinse and refresh the water every 4 hours or so until the little tails appear on the now germinated rice in 24 to 48 hours.
3. When the rice is ready, rinse it several times until it is clean and the water runs clear again.
4. Drain the rinse water and put the rice into a blender or food processor. Add just enough seltzer water to get the rice moving effectively—you don't want it to be too liquefied. This is your base batter and should be very thick and stiff so that it is versatile enough for use in all of the recipes here. Blend until the batter is very smooth. Add more seltzer water if necessary to keep the batter moving.
5. Pour out the batter and freeze any leftover for use in other recipes. Use any frozen batter within a month or two for best results. Simply remove from the freezer and allow it to thaw. Pour off any water that settles to the top for a thicker batter when using with these recipes.

The Arrowroot GABA Galette

The arrowroot galette, based on the humble French galette pastry, is a staple in my kitchen for cannabis tea-time; it's easy to make and can be anything you crave, sweet or savory. Galettes are rustic and roughly hewn—dough can be pressed, filled, and folded by hand in the same pan used for baking it. This arrowroot galette pastry can be a bite, a dessert, or an entire meal when served with salad. I'm going to introduce you to three of my favorite arrowroot galettes in a bit, but what you fill yours with is only limited by your imagination. Galettes like this are often quite good with ingredients you already have on hand, fresh or frozen.

Make the Arrowroot Galette Pastry Dough

¼ cup (60 milliliters) GABA sweet brown rice batter (page 144)
¼ cup (60 milliliters) aquafaba
¼ cup (60 milliliters) coconut oil, or rice bran oil, or olive oil
¼ teaspoon (1 gram) salt
¼ teaspoon (1 gram) baking powder
½ cup (65 grams) arrowroot powder
¾ cup (105 grams) sorghum or ivory teff flour (or a little more, if needed)

This is the basic pastry recipe used to make the galettes featured on the next few pages, or any galette you create with fruits, vegetables, seasonings, or even meat. It makes 1 (6–8-inch or 152–203-millimeter) galette, depending on how thin you roll the crust. Don't press this thinner than a pie crust, approximately one-eighth of an inch (3 millimeters), to ensure that the fillings stay inside of the pastry during baking.

Preparation:

1. Combine the GABA batter, aquafaba, selected oil, and salt. Sweet galettes should be made with either rice bran oil or coconut oil. Savory galettes can be made with any of the oils that pair with the other flavors and ingredients you have selected.

2. In a separate bowl, combine the baking powder, arrowroot, and the sorghum or teff flour. Add a little bit at a time to the wet ingredients while stirring and then work this into a ball. Wrap the dough or cover it so it does not dry out and refrigerate for 15 minutes.

3. Remove the dough from the refrigerator, and roll out or press as you would for a pie crust or press it directly into the pan or plate you will be baking on. Sprinkle with water to keep the dough pliable if needed.

4. Galettes made with this dough will be baked at 350°F (177°C) for 15 to 25 minutes, depending on the filling inside. A gently browned crust and hot filling should indicate doneness in most cases.

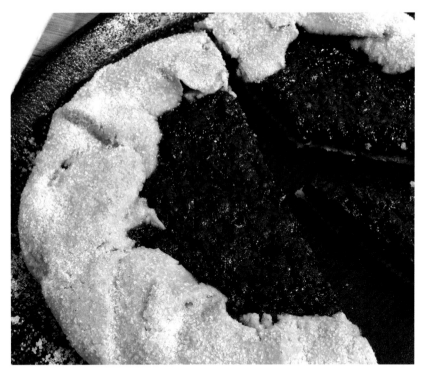

Apricot Rose, Berry Orange Blossom, and Elderberry Galettes

This will make 1 (6–8-inch or 152–203-millimeter) galette based on the dough recipe here.

Apricot Rose

1 rolled out arrowroot galette dough

¾ cup (150 grams) apricots, fresh and sliced

1 tablespoon (8 grams) powdered rose hips

3 tablespoons (45 grams) sugar

2 tablespoons (30 milliliters) culinary rosewater

Additional sugar, for sprinkling generously over the top before baking

---

Berry Orange Blossom

¾ cup (100–130 grams) mixed berries

1 teaspoon (1 gram) arrowroot dissolved in 1 tablespoon (15 milliliters) water mixed in with the berries

3 tablespoons (45 grams)
   sugar
2 teaspoons (10 milliliters)
   orange flower water
Additional sugar, for
   sprinkling generously
   over the top before
   baking

Elderberry
½ rounded cup (80
   grams) elderberries,
   fresh or frozen
½ teaspoon (0.50 grams)
   arrowroot dissolved
   in 2 teaspoons (10
   milliliters) water mixed
   in with the berries
3 tablespoons (45 grams)
   sugar
Additional sugar, for
   sprinkling generously
   over the top before
   baking

Preparation:

1. Preheat the oven to 350°F (177°C) and dust your pastry prep area and baking sheet or pan with a little arrowroot before rolling out the dough.
2. In a small bowl, combine the fruit ingredients as listed. You may also add more sugar to the fruit or for sprinkling on the pastry before baking if you prefer a sweeter pastry.
3. Place your dough on the baking surface and put the filling in the center, working it evenly over the center of the pastry. Fold the pastry around itself and carefully seal the dough around the folded areas to make sure the filling stays inside the pastry. Sprinkle the sugar over the entire top, including the edges.
4. Bake at 350°F (177°C) for about 20 minutes or until the crust is golden and the filling is cooked.
5. Garnish with flowers or terpene entourage for an extra touch!

Lapsang Souchong Smoked Tea and Ham Galette

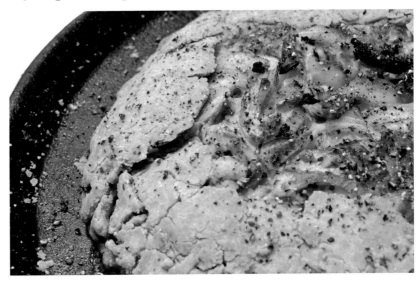

This savory galette is a delicious example of the savory possibilities you have with the Arrowroot GABA Galette. Lapsang Souchong Tea takes the center stage to contribute a deep, smoky flavor to this ham and caramelized onion galette. Makes 1 (6–8-inch or 152–203-millimeter) galette.

1 rolled out arrowroot galette dough (prepared with olive oil)
2 teaspoons (10 milliliters) olive oil
1 medium onion, sliced
1 teaspoon (1 gram) Lapsang Souchong whole tea leaves
Cracked black pepper
Salt, to taste
½ cup (86 grams) uncured ham, sliced into strips
8 or more artichoke heart quarters
1 tablespoon (13 grams) shelled hemp seed
1 garlic clove
¼ teaspoon (1 gram) mustard powder
2 tablespoons (30 milliliters) water

Preparation:

1. Caramelize the sliced onion in 1 teaspoon (5 milliliters) of olive oil and the Lapsang Souchong tea leaves. Crack pepper and salt over this to your liking. Add the sliced ham and briefly stir-fry over the heat, and then transfer to a dish and set aside while preparing the cream sauce.
2. In a blender, add the artichoke hearts, shelled hemp seed, garlic clove, 1 teaspoon (5 milliliters) of olive oil, mustard powder, and a pinch of salt with 1 tablespoon (15 milliliters) of water or a little more, as needed. Blend to turn this into a thick and very smooth sauce.
3. Once you have rolled out the galette, add a thin layer of the onion and ham, followed by the sauce on top of this. Finally, top with the rest of the onion and ham and then fold the galette in, sealing at the bottom as you go along. Crack pepper over the top of the galette.
4. Bake for 25 minutes or more at 350°F (177°C) until golden and bubbly. Allow to rest at least 5 minutes before serving.

Vanilla Cake or Upside-Down Blood Orange Cake with Wild Blackberry Sauce

Quite possibly the best cake you've ever had with a cup of tea! Two recipes in one, this cake is great with any berry sauce, but the wild blackberries that I forage in the summer and fall in California make the best sauce to top this with. This vanilla cake can also be topped with your favorite in-season fruit; the blackberry sauce recipe here is a great template for many fresh fruit toppings! The batter makes terrific cupcakes, too. Makes 1 loaf pan, or 5–7 cupcakes/individual blood orange cakes.

¼ cup (60 milliliters) GABA sweet brown rice batter (page 144)

⅓ cup (80 milliliters) coconut oil

¼ teaspoon (1 gram) salt

¼ teaspoon (1 gram) black salt (kala namak)

¼ cup (60 milliliters) coconut milk

⅔ cup (133 grams) sugar

1 whole vanilla bean, scraped

2 teaspoons (10 milliliters) distilled vinegar

¼ cup (60 milliliters) aquafaba

½ teaspoon (2 grams) baking soda

½ teaspoon (2 grams) baking powder

1¼ cup (176 grams) sorghum or ivory teff flour

⅓ cup (44 grams) + 2 tablespoons (18 grams) arrowroot powder

Optional for Blood Orange Upside-Down Cake

Blood oranges discs, rind removed, thinly sliced

1 tablespoon (15 milliliters) orange flower water

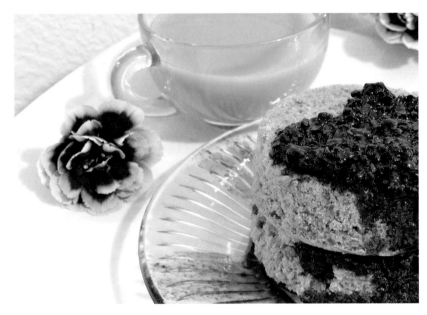

Preparation:

1. Preheat oven to 350°F (177°C), and lightly grease the pan you will be using to bake the cake in with coconut oil and dust it with a little arrowroot powder, if necessary. Set aside. This recipe, like many recipes using the GABA batter and novel grain ingredients of sensitivity cuisine, requires fast work in the kitchen so that the cake rises sufficiently in the oven. You'll want to have your pan greased (if needed), oven heated, and ready to go the minute you have finished mixing and pouring the batter into the pan.

2. Combine the GABA batter, coconut oil, salt, black salt, coconut milk, sugar, scraped vanilla bean, (orange flower water if you are making the Blood Orange Upside-Down Cake), vinegar, and aquafaba in one bowl. Combine the baking powder, baking soda, ivory teff, and arrowroot in

another bowl, and slowly add this to the liquid ingredients in the first bowl and beat until thick, smooth, and very airy.

3. If you're making the Upside-Down Blood Orange Cake, place the orange slices at the bottom of the pan. Spoon the batter evenly into your cake pan or cupcake pan, leaving sufficient space at the top to rise. Bake immediately (don't wait!) for 30 to 35 minutes or until a toothpick comes out clean from the center of the cake.

4. Remove from the oven and let the cake rest on the counter for at least 20 minutes before flipping the pan to release before slicing and topping with berry sauce.

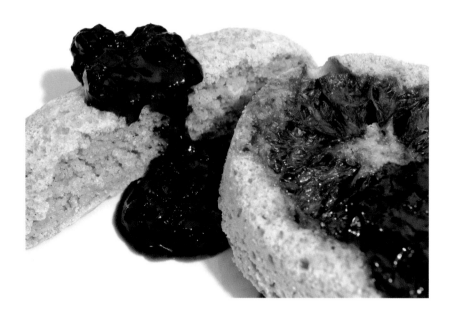

Blackberry Sauce

1½ cups (230 grams) fresh blackberries or other berries

⅓ cup (70 grams) sugar

¼ cup (60 milliliters) water

Preparation:

1. Put everything in a saucepan and simmer until the berry sauce is thick, about 15 minutes or so. Add a little more water, if necessary.
2. Transfer to sauce boat or other serving container. Pour or spoon as much as you'd like over the vanilla or blood orange cake!

Spiced Hemp Banana Bread

¼ cup (60 milliliters) GABA sweet brown rice batter (page 144)

1 large or 2 small/medium overripe bananas, mashed

1 teaspoon (2 grams) chia seed

½ tablespoon (7 milliliters) coconut oil

¼ teaspoon (1 gram) black salt (kala namak)

½ teaspoon (2 grams) salt

⅓ cup (70 grams) sugar

¼ teaspoon (1 gram) cardamom

½ teaspoon (2 grams) cinnamon

1 teaspoon (5 grams) powdered ginger

¼ cup (60 milliliters) seltzer water

½ teaspoon (3 milliliters) vanilla extract

Banana bread has been a sweet staple for breakfast, brunch, and tea-time in American kitchens for more than one hundred years. There are so many ways to make this quick bread—and the spice blend you use can be as

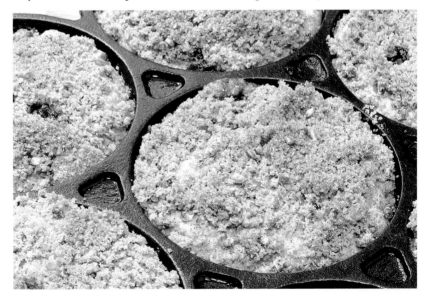

unique as you are! This banana bread features a crunchy topping with whole toasted hemp seeds. Don't confuse these with shelled hemp seed. To get that really special crunch, you need the whole toasted hemp seed. Makes 5–6 muffins or 1 medium loaf of bread.

¼ cup (32 grams) arrowroot powder

1½ cups (180 grams) sorghum flour

1½ teaspoons (7 grams) baking powder

¼ cup (30 grams) berries such as blackberries, blueberries, or elderberries (optional)

For the crunchy toasted hemp seed topping:

1 teaspoon (5 grams) cinnamon

1 tablespoon (8 grams) arrowroot

2 tablespoons (20 grams) sorghum flour

¼ cup (65 grams) brown sugar

1 tablespoon (15 milliliters) coconut oil

1 tablespoon (10 grams) whole toasted hemp seed

Preparation:

1. *For the crumble topping:* Combine all the topping ingredients in a bowl with the oil distributed evenly throughout the topping and set aside.

2. Preheat the oven to 350°F (177°C). Grease your pan with coconut oil, if necessary. In the first bowl, combine the GABA batter, mashed bananas, chia, coconut oil, black salt, salt, sugar, cardamom, cinnamon, ginger, vanilla, and seltzer water. In the second bowl, combine the arrowroot, sorghum flour, and baking powder.

3. Slowly add the dry ingredients to the liquid ingredients until you have a smooth batter. Gently fold in the berries if you have opted to include these in your banana bread.

4. Pour into the pan or muffin tins you have prepared. Evenly distribute the crumbly topping across the top, and bake for 35 minutes or until a toothpick comes out clean when pushed through the center of the bread.

5. Remove from the oven and allow the bread to cool for 15 minutes before serving with your favorite cannabis-infused tea or tisane.

Farmer's Breakfast: Sorghum Biscuits with Sorghum Molasses

Sorghum molasses is produced from the sweet canes of the sorghum plant much the same as tropical sugar cane. But sorghum molasses has a unique flavor that is much lighter, more like honey than the blackstrap molasses produced by sugar cane.

This farmer's breakfast is no leisurely affair—it will have your stiff joints moving and give you an energetic lift that is exactly what you need before laboring in your own cannabis garden this morning!

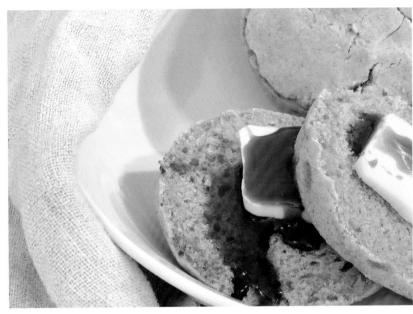

⅓ cup (80 milliliters) GABA sweet brown rice batter (page 144)

2 tablespoons (30 milliliters) coconut oil

½ teaspoon (2 grams) salt

¼ cup (60 milliliters) seltzer water

2 tablespoons (30 milliliters) whole cream coconut milk

3 tablespoons (45 milliliters) aquafaba

1½ teaspoons (6 grams) baking powder

1 cup (140 grams) sorghum flour

⅓ cup (44 grams) arrowroot powder

Your desired breakfast beverage infused with cannabis should be prepared right before hot biscuits are served with your choice of butter or coconut oil. These biscuits are also delicious when smothered with a savory sausage gravy or a sweet option like sorghum molasses—you could also place both gravy and molasses with the biscuits and let your guests choose which they'd rather. Makes about 6 medium-sized biscuits. Double or triple the recipe for more.

Preparation:

1. Preheat the oven to 360°F (182°C) and grease a biscuit pan or other baking pan with coconut oil, if necessary.

2. In the first bowl, combine the GABA batter, coconut oil, salt, seltzer water, coconut milk, and aquafaba. In a second bowl, combine the baking powder, sorghum flour, and arrowroot powder. Add the dry

ingredients to the liquid ingredients slowly while stirring until you have a soft biscuit dough that can be spooned or shaped into biscuit size. Add more seltzer water if you need more moisture in the dough.

3. Bake for 15 minutes or until golden on top. Remove from oven and allow these to cool briefly before serving with sorghum molasses or gravy. Can be reheated and served any time of the day.

The GABA Fry

Let's be honest here: when you consume cannabis, it's easy and way too much fun to indulge in fried foods and other naughty food treats. But fried foods don't have to be "junky" when you make them at home with nutritious oils, fresh vegetables and proteins, and my special whole grain GABA Fry coating. GABA Fry is always a favorite indulgence of mine and of guests in my home and pairs beautifully with iced cannabis teas.

The GABA Fry is everything you need in terrific crunch and flavor to satisfy the munchies. This fry method has the distinct advantage of crisping again upon reheating, as well. It's sure to become your favorite fry method!

Make the Batter and Dredge

The basic batter and dredge recipe is very plain—salt only. Seasonings and dipping sauces are prepared individually for the kind of fry you want to create. The coating batter is always the same: ½ cup (120 milliliters) GABA batter and enough aquafaba added to make it the same consistency as pancake batter, typically 1 tablespoon (15 milliliters) or so, if needed.

The dredge is an arrowroot-rich flour coating, and this is where all of your salt and seasonings will go. You will dredge whatever you want to fry after coating it in the batter in a mixture of ½ cup (65 grams) arrowroot powder and ½ cup (80 grams) of either ivory teff or sorghum flour plus all of the desired seasonings.

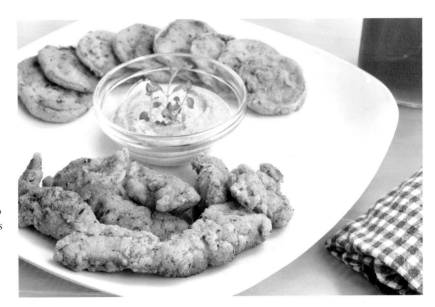

Fry Ingredients
Rice bran oil, for frying
Chicken breast, sliced into
fingers or nugget pieces
Whole green tomatoes,
sliced into rounds

Dredge Seasoning
2 teaspoons (3 grams)
thyme or lemon thyme
1 teaspoon (4 grams) salt
1 teaspoon (2 grams)
black pepper
½ teaspoon (1 gram)
garlic powder
½ teaspoon (1 gram)
onion powder
½ teaspoon (1 gram)
white pepper
½ teaspoon (1 gram)
cayenne pepper
½ teaspoon (1 gram)
smoked paprika

Southern Sweetie Cannabis Sweet Tea + Crispy Cajun Chicken & Fried Green Tomato Bites

Fried green tomatoes are among my favorite fry cuisine. They always get a lot of raves from guests—who always ask for the recipe. This fry uses rice bran oil because of its neutral flavor and the wonderful crisp it gives to both the chicken fingers and green tomatoes.

Brew the sweet tea very concentrated using black or Pekoe tea. When the tea is finished brewing, sweeten it, and whisk the cannabis infusion of your choice from the introductory chapter into the warm tea. Refrigerate to cool while you prepare the chicken and green tomatoes. Whisk the tea vigorously before pouring over ice and serving.

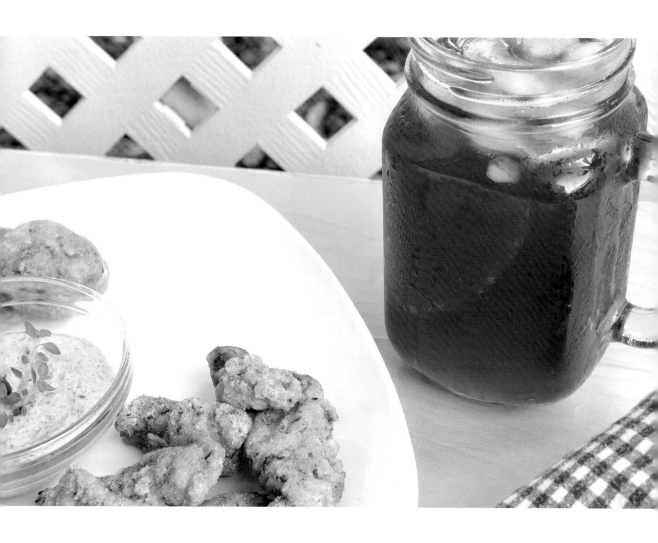

Preparation:

1. Preheat the rice bran oil in your frying pan.
2. Coat the chicken and tomato slices in the GABA batter and then dredge through the flour and seasoning mixture.
3. Fry until golden brown on all sides. Drain and serve with hot sauce or your favorite dipping sauce.

Mediterranean Minty Canna–Tea + Fried Artichoke Hearts and Lemon Bites

Fry Ingredients
Olive oil, for frying
Frozen or canned artichoke hearts, quartered
1 whole lemon, thinly sliced

Dredge Seasoning:
1 teaspoon (4 grams) salt
1 teaspoon (2 grams) black pepper
1 teaspoon (2 grams) dried Greek oregano
1 teaspoon (1 gram) thyme
½ teaspoon (1 gram) cumin
½ teaspoon (1 gram) sumac

Brew the Mediterranean mint tea with half Gunpowder green tea and half spearmint leaves, lemon balm leaves, and lavender flowers. When your tea has finished brewing and is still hot, add the cannabis infusion of your choice from the introductory chapter. Refrigerate and allow to cool to room temperature. Whisk vigorously before pouring over ice and serving with the artichoke and lemon bites.

Preparation:

1. Preheat the olive oil in your frying pan.
2. Coat the artichoke hearts and lemon slices in the GABA batter and then dredge through the flour and seasoning mixture.
3. Fry until golden brown on all sides. Drain and serve.

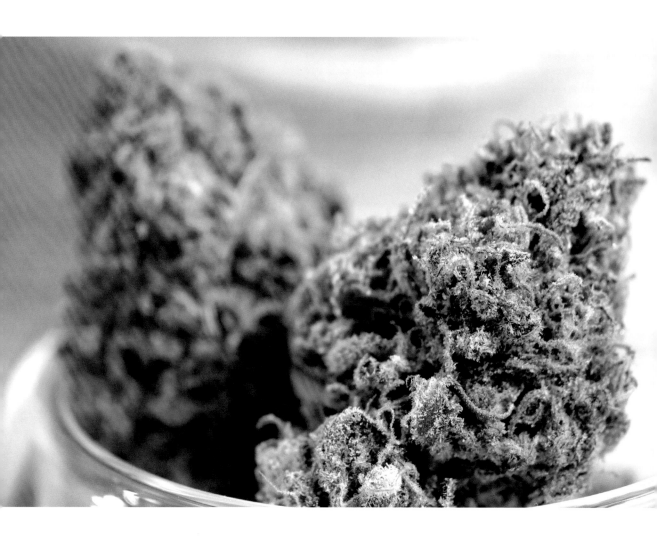

CONCLUSION AND RESOURCE GUIDE

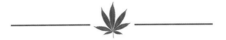

You are now ready to create your own cannabis-tea time tradition at home, for holidays or any special event! It's time to start thinking about stocking your kitchen or creating a tea-nook for your special cannabis tea-time every day. This resource guide is a list of reputable retailers of the many fine ingredients that are in this book—this is my personal list and where I shop most frequently. —*Sandra*

Lekithos Inc. / mysunflowerlecithin.com
Lekithos is a solvent-free and GMO-free sunflower lecithin I use and recommend.

Amazon and Vitacost / amazon.com / vitacost.com
Two great online stores that offer free shipping for grocery items, ivory teff, sorghum, teas, sweet brown rice, and specialty oils. You'll find almost everything you need to make the recipes in this book at reasonable prices.

Mei Leaf Tea / meileaf.com
Don Mei, one of the most respected tea merchants in the UK has a fabulous store where you can order the best teas in the world! And if you are visiting London you will want to stop by his shop for a memorable Gong Fu tea experience too.

Red Rose Tea Classic and Arabic Lipton Yellow Label

These are two commercial-grade bagged teas that I am not ashamed to recommend to even the most discriminating of tea geeks. I don't usually do bagged teas, but when I do, it's one or both of these brands. Red Rose is going to be easier to find than the authentic Arabic Lipton Yellow Label—Walmart typically carries Red Rose Classic while ethnic grocers will most often carry the Arabic Lipton Yellow Label. Note that the Arabic Lipton Yellow Label is very different in flavor and body from the typical Lipton tea brand most commonly sold in the West. Do not substitute Western Lipton for Arabic Lipton, use Red Rose instead.

Adagio Teas, Tea Trekker, Silk Road Teas / adagio.com / teatrekker.com / silkroadteas.com

I order my tea from these stores and have been impressed with the quality. Tea Trekker is one of the few tea stores that reliably carries authentic milk oolong. You may also take advantage of $15 off of your first order at Silk Road Teas by going here: http://r.sloyalty.com/r/vrr0T11mL58C

Spicely / spicely.com

My favorite spice store—everything they stock is authentic and very fresh.

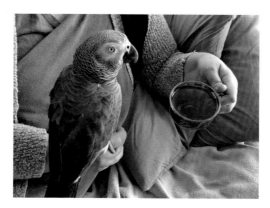

INDEX

tea infusion of, 112
tea service for, 39, 45
terpenes of, 1, 9, 41–44, 53, 55–58, 62, 71, 76–78, 82, 84–88, 91, 94–95, 97–98, 125, 138–140, 143
tinctures of, 3
trim of, 8
Canned beans
aquafaba and, 137, 139
chickpeas, 137
white beans, 137
Carcinogenic, 82–83
Cardamom
brown, 109
green, 109, 129
Carnation
petals of, 32
Carrots, 97–98, 100–101
Caryophyllene, 44, 49, 93
Caster sugar, 45–49, 57, 91
Caster xylitol, 45, 47–49
Cayenne pepper, 132, 157
CBD
oil of, 86
Celery, 97–98, 100, 135
Ceramic tea pets, 25–26
Ceylon cinnamon sticks, 110
Ceylon tea, 122
Chahai, 24
Chai tea, 109–121
Chamomile, 46, 86
Cheesecloth, 48, 69–70, 79, 95, 106–107, 116–117
Cherry, 114–117, 119, 131, 133

Cherry Syrup, 116–117, 119
Chia, 153–154
Chicken
broth and, 97–98
carcass of, 96–98
fried, 157
Chickpeas, 137
Chili
pods of, 98
powder of, 93
China, 22
Chocolate, 131–132
Cholesterol, 14
Chronic pain, 11
Cilantro, 102
Cinnamon sticks
Ceylon, 110
Citron. 32, 44, 71, 79–80, 129, 136
Citrus
blossom of, 46, 84, 127
fruit of, 76, 129
peels of, 46
Clarity
beverage and, 22
broth and, 33
Clay dish, 24–25, 28
Clear sinuses, 82
Clinical studies, 12
Clove, 44, 46, 97–102, 109, 129, 150
CO2
cannabis extractions and, 13
Coconut
flavor of, 14

ice cream, 132–133
milk of, 105–110, 112, 119, 121–123, 127, 151, 155
oil of, 13–14, 16, 18, 139–142, 147, 151, 153–155
Colds, 81, 97
Cookie cutter, 140
Cracked pepper, 100, 143
Cracker, 141–142
Crema, 57–58
Cross-contact
food preparation and, 105
Culinary
Styles, 135
Cumin, 102, 159
Curing process
blackberry leaves and, 74–75
wild olives and, 78
Curry, 47, 93

D

Dairy, 55, 105, 132–133, 135
Dairy flavorings
milk oolong and, 55
Dairy-free, 132–133
Damascenone, 49, 93
DEA, 82
Decarboxylate
cannabinoids and, 3, 17–18, 38
Dedicated factory
food production and, 13–14
Dehydration
fruits and, 74
herbs and, 74

sun and, 73–74
Dessert beverages, 6, 33, 108, 110
Distilled vinegar, 47–48, 92, 151
Distilled water , 46, 48–49, 92
Doctors, 15, 66–69, 136
Dong Quai, 96
Dosage
    calculation of, 8, 17, 19, 38
Dr. Leary, 41
Dr. Sanjay Gupta, 43
Dredge
    frying, and, 156
Drowsiness, 10
Dry salt cure, 78
Drying plate or rack, 45

E
Eggs
    whites, of, 46
    structures, like, 137
Elderberry
    European species of, 81
    flowers of, 75–76
    fruit of, 32, 80–81
    west coast species of, 80–81
Electric dehydration, 73–74
Elizabeth Bird, 136
Emerald Triangle, 132–133
Emulsifiable infusion oil
    cannabis and, 16
Emulsification
    liquids and, 3, 20
Energizing, 44, 79, 102
Entourage effect, 43
Entourage tea

method of, 41
    terpenes and, 42–53
Environmental humidity, 45
Essential oils, 42, 48, 53, 82, 91
Eucalyptus, 82
Europe , 67, 72, 81, 110
Eyedropper, 16, 18, 25

F
Fan brush
    culinary use of, 47
Farmer's markets, 137
Fatigue-fighter, 79
Fats
    beverage and, 3, 12–13
    solvents of, 3
FDA, 82
Fennel
    bulb, 101
    flowers, 87, 100–101
    pollen, 101
    seeds, 102, 109
Fiber, 20, 35, 47, 106–107
Fine detail brush
    culinary use of, 47
Fish
    allergies and, 135
Flatbread, 141
Flours, 137, 139, 141, 144,
    146–147, 151, 154–156, 159
Flu, 97
Food dehydrator, 48
Foraging, 68
Formal
    tea service and, 22, 39

Fragrance, 15–16, 18, 22, 25–26,
    29, 42, 48, 50, 62, 74, 82–83,
    114–115, 117
France
    culinary herb blend, of
Fresh flowers
    basil, 44, 46, 49, 93, 100
    blackberry, 32, 46, 49, 72–77,
        81, 84, 87, 121, 133, 150,
        153
    chamomile, 46, 86
    carnation, 32, 44, 46
    cherry, 46, 114–117, 119, 133
    citrus, 43, 46, 76, 84, 87–88,
        97, 127, 129
    rose, 32, 42, 46, 49–50, 53,
        58, 62, 84, 87, 93, 125,
        138–139
    terpene entourage and, 45–53
    violet, 46
Fried green tomatoes, 157
Fruits
    apricot, 32, 148
    apple, 32, 62
    banana, 153–154
    blood orange, 49, 76–77,
        150–153
    Buddha's hand citron, 129
    lime, 47–50, 92–93
    lemon, 22, 32, 42–44, 46–53,
        71, 80, 82, 91–93, 97–98.
        102, 159
    rose hips, 148
    terpene entourage and, 45–53
Fujian jasmine pearl tea, 30